Acup  Moxibustion in the Treatment of Irritable Bowel Syndrome

A Narrative Review

By John Cassone, PhD, LAc, DAOM

Dr. Cassone

Dr. Cassone

Dr. Cassone

ACKNOWLEDGEMENTS

I have enjoyed a rich academic experience in my years at South Baylo University completing the Masters program and now the Doctoral program. I am grateful for the high quality professors and doctors that have shaped my understanding of this amazing medicine. In particular, I would like to thank Dr. Sandjaya Trikadibusana for giving me, with patience, many classroom and clinic hours of wisdom. Dr. Trikadibusana has made a tremendous impact on me both personally and professionally. I often keep him in mind as I treat patients in my own clinic.

I would like to thank Dr. Wayne Cheng for the many hours of encouragement and support given during the entire doctoral program at South Baylo University. At the end of the Masters program, he encouraged me to start the Doctoral program and remained a strong student advocate during the entire program. I have spent countless hours in his office and feel grateful for his guidance. He is the reason I kept my sanity and the reason I was able to complete the DAOM.

Dr. Cassone

DEDICATION

My greatest accomplishments are built on the greatest support. There's nothing I do that doesn't include a tremendous amount of care, support, encouragement, and love from my favorite person, Kelly Cassone. This work, in my pursuit of academic and professional excellence, is dedicated to her.

Dr. Cassone

The Effectiveness of Acupuncture and Moxibustion in the Treatment of Irritable Bowel Syndrome

A Narrative Review

John Cassone

SOUTH BAYLO UNIVERSITY at ANAHEIM, 2018

Research Advisor: Sandjaya Trikadibusana, L.Ac., Ph.D., M.D.

Dr. Cassone

ABSTRACT

Diseases and disorders of the gastrointestinal tract are common and increasing in the developed world. Irritable bowel syndrome (IBS) is one of such disorders which comes with a high morbidity rate. Conventional care models are branch treatment focused, meaning they interrupt the disease mechanism but do not address the cause of the disease. They do not treat by improving normal function or identifying factors that disrupt function and are also associated with high costs and undesirable side effects. According to the National Center for Complementary and Integrative Health, acupuncture is considered safe with relatively few complications. The purpose of this study is to review current research on the treatment of IBS, and the related symptoms of visceral hyperalgesia, using acupuncture and moxibustion applied to specific acupoints. A narrative review was conducted by performing a comprehensive search on four electronic databases: the Cochrane Central Register of Controlled Trials, PubMed, Alt Health Watch, and EBSCO, and the following keywords were used; "irritable bowel syndrome and acupuncture," "irritable bowel syndrome and moxibustion," "visceral hypersensitivity and acupuncture," and "visceral hypersensitivity and moxibustion." Studies more than 5 years old, opinion based articles (including blog entries), and all non-scientific or non-peer reviewed articles were excluded. Studies involving laser acupuncture, acupressure, auricular acupuncture, ear seeds, or reflexology were also excluded. From the 26 articles yielded there were 3 systematic reviews, 3 qualitative reviews, 1 case study, 11 RCTs using animal subjects, and 8 RCTs using human subjects. The results of the review showed evidence for the effectiveness in treating IBS related symptoms with a variety of measurable outcomes using multiple acupuncture and moxibustion treatment strategies. While there is significant evidence that acupuncture and moxibustion can positively affect factors and symptoms related to IBS, more thorough and well-designed Randomized and Controlled Trials are needed for mainstream medical acceptance.

TABLE OF CONTENTS

Dr. Cassone

INTRODUCTION

Irritable Bowel Syndrome (IBS) refers to a set of symptoms primarily affecting the gastrointestinal system. According to the National Institute for Diabetes and Digestive and Kidney Diseases, it is estimated that 15% of the population in the developed world suffers IBS. Chronic IBS has affected 26.9% of adults in the United States with an increased economic burden (Sandler, Stuart, and Liberman, 2010). The total cost of IBS is estimated $200 billion worldwide (McFarland, 2008). The general prevalence of IBS around the world is approximately 11% (Hungin, 2003) with the majority being adult females (Lovell and Ford, 2012). The primary symptoms include cramping, pain, gas, constipation alternating with loose stool, sense of urgency to defecate, distention of the lower abdomen, and poor appetite.

Within the conventional medical care umbrella, the cause of IBS is viewed to be unknown and incurable although the onset is closely related to psychological stress (Drossma, Camerilli, and Mayer, 2002). IBS occurs more often in high stress work environments (Pan, Lu, & Ke, 2000) and has a greater frequency in women than men (Grundmann & Yoon, 2010). IBS is considered to be a diagnosis of exclusion as most patients present without inflammatory, anatomic, metabolic, or neoplastic factors to define the etiology and pathophysiology. For a disease to be defined through diagnosis there must be objectively measurable abnormalities. If examinations do not reveal measurable and objective disease indications, then the condition is regarded as a functional illness or syndrome, in which case treatment is either not offered or it is only aimed at symptom relief. Drugs aimed at symptom relief do not stop the condition or prevent it from worsening. These drugs also cause undesirable side effects. Once the symptoms progress to the state of a measurable disease, treatment becomes based on interruption of the disease mechanism. For example using antibiotics to treat an infection, which was caused by poor gut health, without improving the gut health. Assessment of digestive system functions related to pathology, and treatment to improve normal function, is not currently covered in conventional care approaches.

Over the last few years, the modern field of medicine has regained a sense of importance to the gastrointestinal system as it relates to the physiologies and pathologies of the rest of the body. Although other medical modalities, such as Acupuncture and Oriental Medicine (AOM), often view systemic patterns of disease as having started in the gut, it is a relatively new trend in conventional care. Terms such as "leaky gut" for the first time are being used to connect the digestive system to disorders such as depression, anxiety, headaches, allergies, acne, eczema, arthritis, fibromyalgia, and other chronic states of inflammation as well as autoimmune disorders. The need for care models aimed at treating the functions of the gastrointestinal system and restoring its normal physiology is at an all-time high. This window of opportunity is what makes the timing and topic of this research relevant and important.

In AOM, which uses acupuncture and moxibustion for treatment, the function of the system and the disease of the system are inseparable. Pathogenesis is described based on how the functional problem results in the disease pattern. The acupuncture and moxibustion approach to treatment intrinsically includes the restoration of function that originally caused the disease. It is only by treating the cause, or the root of a condition, that long term health can be restored.
There are many studies on the use of acupuncture in the treatment of IBS. This review is significant because of the

timing in public awareness and consumer demand, medical trends regarding gastrointestinal health, and time period of research data collected. This review only includes studies within the last five years and it includes studies using moxibustion, which are not as common as acupuncture studies. The purpose of this review is to analyze current research studies, including treatment strategies when possible, and present evidence that the combination of acupuncture and moxibustion is a valid and effective treatment option for patients suffering IBS.

REVIEW OF LITERATURE

Western Medicine Viewpoint:

Conventional Diagnosis and Treatment

IBS is broken into subcategories based on the prevailing stool pattern: constipation (IBS-C), diarrhea (IBS-D), mixed constipation and diarrhea (IBS-M), or unsubtyped (IBS-U). Gut dysmotility may also be broken down into four sub-groups: spastic colon syndrome, functional diarrhea, diarrhea-predominant spastic colon syndrome, and midgut dysmotility (Cole, Duncan, & Claydon, 2002). Causative factors for IBS are highly variable and complex and a single pathogenesis has not been identified. Most studies indicate that IBS is associated with visceral hypersensitivity, disruption in gut motility, and abnormal function of the gut-brain axis. Visceral hypersensitivity, and visceral hyperalgesia, are terms used to characterize the internal pain of organs (viscera), in this case specifically describing pain within the gastrointestinal tract. Visceral hypersensitivity, as a benchmark for IBS severity, is used to gauge the progression and remission of IBS (Nozu, Okumura, 2011) as it appears to be the main underlying cause of the abdominal pain symptoms in patients with IBS (Keszthelyi, Troost, & Masclee, 2012). Chronic visceral hypersensitivity involves the brain-gut axis and can manifest in the spinal cord, the periphery, and the central nervous system (Kang, Jia, 2008). The brain-gut axis can affect the outer periphery, the spinal cord, the central nervous system, and various associated neurotransmitters (Weng, 2015). The enteric nervous system is affiliated with the central nervous system, which regulates gastrointestinal function, while the reciprocal relationships are referred to as brain-gut interactions (Kim and Camilleri, 2000). When attempting to induce bowel sensitivity in patients, through colonic irrigation, the patients suffering IBS show significantly lower pain thresholds compared to healthy patients, which illustrates the visceral hypersensitivity component of IBS (Dong, 2004). Visceral hypersensitivity can be used to differentiate IBS-D from Functional Diarrhea. Although the two ailments present with a similar set of symptoms, only IBS-D presents with abdominal pain that is improved with defecation (Camerilleri, Sellin, and Barrett, 2016).

Conventional Diagnostics and Differential Diagnoses

Comprehensive stool analysis can identify parasites, fungus, and other infections that need to be ruled out. Helicobactor pylori infections are common and, if discovered, will be treated with a triple antibiotic cocktail; however, this approach causes further damage to the integrity of the gut microbiome, which consequently increases the recurrence rate of infections. Celiac disease must also be excluded when there is severe irritation to the gastrointestinal system. A Positive test will help to eliminate a major dietary cause (gluten containing foods). Endoscopic images are used to rule out pathologies of the upper gastrointestinal tract such as Barrett's Esophagitis, stomach cancers, gastritis, herniations, ulcers, stenosis, or other visual structure abnormalities. Treatment of upper gastrointestinal tract disorders includes drugs and surgeries. Pancreatic enzymes can be evaluated to rule out pancreatitis, tumors of the pancreas, or diabetic pathologies. Hydrogen breath tests can be used to screen for fruit or lactose malabsorption (in which case, those foods are removed from the diet). Blood tests will show immune system involvement and liver enzyme abnormalities. Colonoscopy images are used to rule out cancers of the colon, diverticulitis, polyps, ulcerations, or structural changes. Biopsies are taken as needed to rule out oncogenesis.

Ultrasound equipment is used to check for gallbladder related conditions such as gallstones. If the gallbladder is congested or has stones it will be surgically removed. These differential diagnoses only tell a doctor what the patient does not have. The benefit of exhaustive tests is early detection of time sensitive disease patterns, such as cancer. The downside of these approaches, as they relate to IBS, is that patients end up waiting to get worse before more diagnosable aspects of the disorder manifest.

When a diagnosis of IBS has been given, an MD may prescribe psychiatric medications to reduce stress and anxiety. Visceral hypersensitivity correlates to elevations in stress which affect the brain-gut axis (Whitehead, Palsson, 1998). Laxatives are prescribed for IBS-C, while antacids in the form of proton pump inhibitors or H2 antagonists are prescribed generally for any form of indigestion related to IBS. Anticholinergics, antimotility drugs, and antidiarrheal agents are prescribed for patients with IBS-D (Abdullah and Firmansyah, 2013); however, these drugs also have side effects ranging from drowsiness, abdominal pain, distention, dizziness, nausea, vomiting, constipation, dependency, tolerance, and respiratory depression (Mangel, Bornstein, and Hamm, 2008).

Additional Western Science Concepts Related to IBS

Purinergic P2X receptors transmit pain signals (Loguercio, 2012). When the intestinal lumen is expanded, adenosine triphosphate (ATP) is released. The P2X receptors open when they bind with extracellular ATP. The stimulus resulting from the stretching triggers the nerve plexus with the P2X receptor located within the mucosal lining, which transmits pain signals to the brain (Burnstock and Kennedy, 2011). When lumenal nociceptors are inflamed they send afferent nerve impulses through dorsal root ganglia (DRG). This triggers a response in the central nervous system (Blackshaw, Brookes, & Grundy, 2007). The P2X receptors generate action potentials (Rong, Spider, & Burnstock, 2002) which means they play a major role in pain signaling for IBS patients. Recurrent hyper-distention of the intestinal lumen results in hyperexcitability of the sensory neurons, and of the central nervous system, which triggers spasms and cramps in the intestines (Shinoda, Feng, & Gebhart, 2009). P2X receptors are crucial in the inflammatory and pain cycles, which is why they are often targets for anti-inflammation and anti-nociception drugs (Kong, Liu, & Xu, 2013).

ATP regulates pain signals by binding to the P2X receptors (Giniatullin and Nistri, 2013), and is also is involved in other IBS related functions such as intestinal motility and gastrointestinal secretions. ATP is held in intestinal secretory cells and transfer signals from peripheral sensory neurons (Tamir, Gershon, 1990). ATP communicates intercellular signals through purinergic receptors (Burnstock, 1997), these signals are introduced to the spinal cord through the dorsal root ganglion, and go to the brainstem via interneurons, which involve the motor neurons of the gastrointestinal tract. Signals are also sent to the pain area of the cerebral cortex to decrease sensation of pain (Zhao, 2008).

The pain relieving mechanism of acupuncture may be due to the binding of adenosine triphosphate (ATP) with purinergic receptors of sensory nerve endings of the skin, which induces a signal conduction pathway for pain modulation in the cerebral cortex. P2X receptors are located throughout the entire body and play a major role in neuropathic, inflammatory, and visceral pain (Xu, Shenoy, and Winston, 2008). Therefore, when reviewing studies involving the treatment of IBS, it is useful to keep in mind the relationship between the P2X receptor and IBS visceral hypersensitivity within the biological feedback loop of the brain-gut axis. In the central nervous system, P2X receptors influence synaptic plasticity and balance neurotransmitters of the dorsal horn in the spinal cord. The P2X receptors of the dorsal root ganglion (DRG) affect sensory neurons and are important in treating ATP-mediated pain in IBS patients (Shinoda, La, & Bielefeldt, 2010).

Brain imaging in patients suffering IBS appears uniquely compared to healthy patients (Elsenbruch, Rosenburg, & Bingel, 2010). IBS patients show distinctly different visceral sensory areas of the brain from healthy populations (Mertz, Morgan, & Tanner, 2000). IBS patients also show changes in blood circulation, carbohydrate metabolism, and processes of the cerebral cortex (Ringel, Drossman, & Turkington, 2003). Rectal irritation through distention has been shown to provoke the anterior cingulate cortex, prefrontal cortex, inferior colliculus, and thalamus (Mertz, Morgan, & Tanner, 2000) illustrating the gut-brain axis. IBS patients display increased dorsolateral prefrontal cortex activity compared to normosensitive patients (Larsson, Tillisch, & Craif, 2012). Brain-gut peptides also modulate gastrointestinal functions and are an important influence on IBS patterns. Excitatory neurotransmitters include histamine, 5-HT, substance P, calcitonin gene-related peptide, and corticotropin-releasing factor-related peptide, while inhibitory neurotransmitters include cholecystokinin, norepinephrine, and vasoactive peptide (Gershon, Tack, 2007).

Acupuncture and Oriental Medicine Viewpoint:
Acupuncture and Oriental Medicine Diagnosis and Treatment

Acupuncture and Oriental Medicine (AOM) is a medical model that emphasizes a systems approach to healthcare. Whereas conventional care models view the body as separate parts reductionistically, AOM looks at the big picture holistically. One is not necessarily better than the other in general; however, a systems approach may be more effective, or at least valuable adjunctively, in treating patients with IBS. In China, many doctors consider the AOM approach to be superior to the conventional Western medical approach when treating IBS patients (Tang, 2009). According to AOM, diagnosis is made based on patterns that represent relationships of occurrence within the body which may involve more than one system. For example, IBS is largely considered to be based on one or more of eight core patterns: spleen and stomach qi deficiency, spleen qi deficiency with damp, spleen yang deficiency, kidney yang deficiency, liver qi stagnation, retention of cold damp, retention of damp heat, and retention of food (Anatasi, 2017). Irritable bowel syndrome belongs to the category of disease called diarrhea, constipation, and abdominal pain in Chinese medicine (Zhang, Li, & Wei, 2010); however, treatment will be based on the underlying pattern. The AOM approach also gives a tremendous weight to the emotional state of the patient as possible pathogenesis. Many AOM doctors focus their treatments on the emotional state, with resolution of the emotional state being the primary treatment goal, resulting in improvements in the physical chief complaint. IBS, specifically, is often caused by anxiety or depression (Li, Su, 2011). In IBS patients, the severity of the gastrointestinal symptoms, the level of psychological stress, and abnormal provocation of certain brain regions are related (Drossman, Ringel, & Vogt, 2003). When a patient is no longer stressed, anxious, or depressed then the brain abnormalities connected to visceral hypersensitivity diminish (Chen, Chen, & Yin, 2012). Research supports the evidence that emotional and psychological factors affect IBS which gives reason to emphasize the brain-gut axis. Patients suffering the visceral hypersensitivity of IBS demonstrate increased central reactivity from the outer periphery and also increased visceral sensitivity to central stress events. This further illustrates the brain-gut axis (Fukudo, Nomura, and Muranaka, 1993) and the need for medical models that include emotional and psychological factors in the diagnosis and treatment of IBS. However, most research design leaves no room for individual emotional states to be assessed or considered. This is a core limitation when attempting to justify AOM treatments through Western Science validation.

Moxibustion is a form of AOM treatment using the dried leaves of the herb mugwort (Artemisia vulgaris) burned over acupoints. Its therapeutic effect comes from the thermal stimulation combined with the warming and blood moving qualities of the herb. Although the precise mechanisms are unclear, moxibustion benefits come primarily from its thermal effects (Lee, Kang, 2010). The ability to generate these thermal effects varies based on the quality of the herb used, the size and volume of the moxa cone, and the number of cones applied. There are two primary types of moxa, direct and indirect. Direct moxa is applied directly to the skin whereas indirect moxibustion is applied from a distance to the skin or through an herbal barrier to the skin which can give an additional therapeutic element (e.g. aconite). Moxa also has an important effect on mast cells in the gastrointestinal tract. The number of mast cells, and rate of infiltration and degranulation, are elevated in IBS patients compared to normosensitive patients (Park, Rhee, & Kim, 2006). Moxa stimulates a histamine response that amplifies the effect of mast cells (Pan, Guo, 2009). Moxibustion causes mast cells to degranulate and produce bioactive substances that improve capillary permeability which increases movement of tissue fluid. Moxibustion can increase the number, distribution area, and degranulation of mast cells (Luo, He, & Guo, 2007) which makes it, theoretically, an important treatment for patients suffering IBS.

Acupuncture involves the insertion of sterile stainless steel needles into the body for the purpose of stimulating a healing response in the body. The mechanism of action is controversial as it may involve multiple systems. Acupuncture treatments involve the central nervous system, autonomic nervous system, and enteric nervous system (Li, Zhu, and Rong, 2007). Regarding IBS, intestinal motility is at least partially mediated by neural and humoral pathways which acupuncture can influence. Acupuncture also affects serotonergic, cholinergic, and glutaminergic pathways within the brain-gut axis (Schneider, Weiland, & Enck, 2007) which gives us clues to its global or holistic applications. The use of acupuncture targeting serotonergic, cholinergic, and glutamatergic pathways in IBS patients can, theoretically, stimulate endogenous opioids which decrease visceral pain (Ma, Tan, & Yang, 2009). In general, the response acupuncture generates is a subject of much debate; however, it is the aim of this review to capture credibility and efficacy scientifically, regardless of the precise mechanism of function. In China, acupuncture is considered to be effective in the treatment gastrointestinal diseases (Zheng and Zhang, 2016); however, in the United States it is under utilized. Electroacupuncture (EA) is a technique that adds electrical impulse to acupuncture points. It is effective in alleviating both sensory and inflammatory pain (Zhang, Lao, Ren, and Berman, 2014), including the visceral neuropathic pain in IBS patients (Ji, Li, Lin, 2014). QOL scores improve significantly in patients with gastrointestinal diseases when they are treated with acupuncture (Zhang, Yu, and Xu, 2013).

MATERIALS AND METHODS

Literature Search Strategy

Four electronic databases were used for literature selection: the Cochrane Central Register of Controlled Trials, PubMed, Alt Health Watch, and EBSCO. A comprehensive search of databases was executed using the keywords "irritable bowel syndrome and acupuncture," "irritable bowel syndrome and moxibustion," "visceral hypersensitivity and acupuncture," and "visceral hypersensitivity and moxibustion."

The initial search yielded 322 total articles. Many articles that came up in the search had no relevance to acupuncture or moxibustion. From an initial scan on articles and abstracts, 201 were eliminated based on subject relevance. Duplicates were also eliminated. Of the remaining 125 articles, 36 we unavailable in full text. 29 other article were eliminated because they did not involve acupuncture or moxibustion or IBS. Of the remaining 60 articles, 26 were not available in English. Of the remaining 34 articles, 6 were only proposals for future RCTs and did not include study results. A final total of 26 articles were identified and chosen for this review. Of the 26 articles yielded, there were 3 systematic reviews, 3 qualitative reviews, 1 case study, 11 RCTs using animal subjects, and 8 RCTs human subjects. See figure 1 for a summary of the selection process.

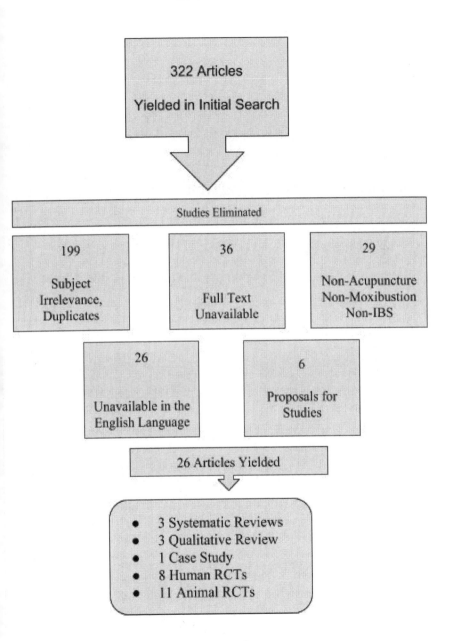

Figure 1. Article selection flow chart

Inclusion Criteria

The types of studies that were allowed in the search process included RCTs, uncontrolled clinical trials, prospective case studies, systematic/meta-analysis reviews, literature reviews, and qualitative studies. Only English language studies were included. There was no discernment made between manual acupuncture, electroacupuncture, direct moxibustion, and indirect moxibustion. In summary, the inclusion criteria were studies performed between January 2012 and December 2017, studies reported in full text English articles that were peer reviewed and studies involving subjects that were treated with acupuncture or moxibustion for IBS related symptoms.

Exclusion Criteria

Studies more than 5 years old were excluded. Opinion based articles, including blog entries, and all non-scientific or non-peer reviewed articles were excluded. Studies without full text availability were excluded. Studies involving laser acupuncture, acupressure, auricular acupuncture, ear seeds, or reflexology were excluded. In summary, the exclusion criteria were studies older than five years, studies not in the English language, laser acupuncture, ear seeds, reflexology, and acupressure. Studies involving other ailments of the gastrointestinal tract were also excluded if they did not included IBS symptomatology.

Study Evaluations

The study design is a narrative review. Based on the exclusion and inclusion criteria, full texts of eligible studies were obtained from one of the four aforementioned databases and reviewed. They were categorized based on their study types: RCTs, systematic reviews/meta-analyses, case studies, and qualitative studies. The data from the studies were extracted and compared. The following items were extracted: author(s), study design, number of subjects, publication year, outcome measurements, and major results.

Randomized Controlled Trials (Human Subjects)

Clinical Study #1

MacPherson et al. (2016)performed a randomized controlled trial to study the use of acupuncture in the treatment of irritable bowel syndrome at 12 months post-randomization. The aim of the study was to evaluate the effects of acupuncture with patients in primary care with ongoing irritable bowel syndrome. Patients were randomized to an acupuncture group (n=116) that received usual care plus weekly acupuncture treatments for 10 weeks or to a group (n=117) that only received usual care (drug medications). Outcomes were based on a self-reporting scale using the IBS Symptom Severity Score measured at 24 months post randomization. The overall response rate was 61%. The study concluded that there were no statistically significant differences between the acupuncture group and the usual care group at 24 months (p<0.05).

Clinical Study #2

Zhenzhong (2015) conducted a random controlled trial with eighty-five IBS patients randomly divided into electro-acupuncture (EA) and moxibustion (moxa) groups to compare the impacts of EA and moxa on primary gastrointestinal symptoms and the expressions of colonic mucosa-associated neuropeptides substance P (SP) and vasoactive intestinal peptide (VIP). Patients included had either diarrhea-predominant or constipation-predominant irritable bowel syndrome (IBS-D and IBS-C, respectively). ST36 and ST37 were selected as acupoints for electroacupuncture or warm moxibustion treatment once a day for 14 consecutive days. Before and after the treatment sessions, a Visual Analog Pain Scale and the Bristol Stool Form Scale were implemented to evaluate gastrointestinal status. There were 41 participants with IBS-D and 40 with IBS-C that volunteered to receive colonoscopy exams before and after the treatments. During colonoscopy, collections from the sigmoid mucosa were taken to detect SP and VIP expression using immunohistochemistry assay. Both EA and moxa treatments were found to be effective at relieving abdominal pain in IBS-D and IBS-C patients. Moxa was more effective at reducing diarrhea in IBS-D patients, whereas EA was more effective at improving constipation in IBS-C patients. EA and moxa treatments both down-regulated the abnormally increased SP and VIP expression in the colonic mucosa, with no significant difference shown between the two treatments.

Clinical Study #3

Zheng (2016) conducted a randomized and parallel group controlled trial. A total of 448 participants were randomly allocated to 3 electroacupuncture groups and 1 loperamide group in a 1:1:1:1 ratio. These participants recorded weekly diarrhea diaries in a 10-week research period that is composed of a 2-week baseline phase, a 4- week treatment phase, and a 4-week follow-up phase. The diarrhea diaries included such input as stool frequency, stool consistency, normal defecations, and whether special food or drugs for diarrhea were taken. Before being randomized, the participants received baseline evaluations. The participants received 16 sessions of electroacupuncture or oral administration of loperamide daily during the 4-week treatment. Then, the participants were followed up for 4 weeks after treatment. The Bristol score decreased to 5.2 units at the week 4, with an improvement of 0.9 units compared with baseline. The 4 groups were comparable in scores using the Bristol Stool Scale assessed at week 4 and week 8. The study result showed that electroacupuncture was equivalent to loperamide in reducing stool frequency in patients with IBS-D or FD. Additionally, electroacupuncture improved stool consistency, the number of days with normal defecation, and quality of life.

Clinical Study #4

Anatasi (2017) conducted a randomized controlled trial using both moxibustion and acupuncture for the treatment of

IBS. The study was a 24-week three-arm, prospective, parallel groups controlled trial of 171 men and women diagnosed with IBS-D based on Rome III diagnostic criteria for functional gastrointestinal tract disorders. The patients were randomly divided into one of three groups: standard care, individualized care, and sham care. Outcome measurements were based on the reduction of pain and secondary IBS symptoms (e.g bloating, gas, and stool consistency). Subjects were instructed to record their stool patterns using daily journals and took a weekly clinical global impression scale test. The authors of the study attempted to conform to the elements of scientific rigor while maintaining alignment with the foundations of acupuncture and oriental medicine. This study was particularly insightful in contributing eight diagnostic patterns and point prescriptions to cover the spectrum of IBS presentations: spleen and stomach qi deficiency, spleen qi deficiency with damp, spleen yang deficiency, kidney yang deficiency, liver qi stagnation, retention of cold damp, retention of damp heat, and retention of food.

Clinical Study #5

Shi (2015) conducted a randomized parallel controlled study on the effects of electroacupuncture vs the effects of moxibustion therapy for the treatment of irritable bowel syndrome. Eighty two adult IBS patients, ages 18-65 years old, were randomly allocated into two groups (n=41). One group was designated for treatment with moxibustion and the other group was designated for treatment with electroacupuncture. All patients were recruited from the Department of Gastroenterology in Jinhua Municipal Central Hospital between January 2012 and September 2013. Eligibility criteria included patients that displayed symptoms consistent with IBS based on Rome III diagnostic criteria. Baseline and outcome assessments were established based on the Visual Analogue Scale for Irritable Bowel Syndrome (VAS-IBS) to gauge both gastrointestinal symptoms and general well-being. Gastric serotonin secretions were measured using samples from the sigmoid colon. The patients received daily treatments for four consecutive weeks (excluding Sundays). ST25 and ST37 were used bilaterally. A Model LH 100A TENS unit was used to treat the electroacupuncture patients with a stimulation frequency of 2 Hz and intensity of 3.0 mA for 30 minutes. The patients receiving moxibustion were treated for 30 minutes with moxa 2-3 cm above the acupoints with a surface temperature of 46 °C. The results showed a remarkable decline in VAS-IBS total scores in both the EA and moxibustion groups; however, there was no statistical significant difference between the two groups.

Clinical Study #6

A randomized double blind clinical trial was performed in 2014 by Rafiei, Ataie, Ramezani, Etemadi, and Nikyar. 60 patients, between 19 and 61 years in age, that were diagnosed with IBS based on the Rome III diagnostic criteria, were assigned to three groups. 51 were female and 9 were male. Pregnancy, diabetes, autoimmune disorders, and infections of the GI tract were conditions that were excluded in participants. First group received drug therapy, the second group received acupuncture, and the third group received sham acupuncture. The trial started with a 2 week evaluation period before being assigned to the three separate groups. For the acupuncture group, catgut technique was used and applied to UB17, 23, 25, DU3, SP9, 15, ST25, 36, REN12, 4, and KID15. Catgut is a type of cord that is made from the natural fibers of sheep or goat intestine. It is embedded in the acupuncture points to enhance the stimulation for 7-14 days. Catgut implantation is one kind of acupuncture where specific acupuncture points are continuously stimulated. Subjective questionnaires were used to evaluate symptoms, pain, depression and anxiety. The Statistical Package for Social Sciences, version 20, was used to analyze the data. The results showed a significant improvement with the acupuncture group in pain and depression.

Clinical Study #7

A randomized controlled trial was performed by Zhu, Wu, Ma, and Liu in 2014 using moxibustion to relief abdominal pain in patients suffering irritable bowel syndrome. Eighty IBS patients were randomly divided into a moxibustion group and a sham moxibustion group for treatment lasting 4 weeks. Volunteers, 15 patients in the moxibustion group and 13 patients in the sham group, completed two MRI scans during a 50 and 100 ml rectal balloon distention before and after treatment. Rectal pain was assessed with a scan test. The Birmingham IBS Symptom Scale and IBS Quality of Life Scale were used to evaluate the effects of treatment. ST25, REN6, and REN12 were the acupoints chosen for the application of the moxibustion treatment that was applied with an aconite barrier that was 2.5 cm diameter. Treatments were applied 3 times per week for duration of 2 weeks. The results showed a statistically significant decrease in symptoms in the moxibustion group. The moxa group also showed improvements in the prefrontal cortex, while the prefrontal cortex and the anterior cingulated cortex were affected in the control group. During the 100 ml distention before treatments in both groups, the prefrontal cortex and the anterior cingulated cortex were provoked. After treatment, the effect reduced in the moxibustion group but remained in the sham group. The research group concluded that moxibustion can improve the symptoms and quality of life in patients suffering IBS by decreasing rectal sensitivity.

Clinical Study #8

In 2014, Zhao, Wu, and Liu performed a factorial study to examine the effects of aconite-separated moxibustion. A total of 166 IBS patients, between the ages of 18 and 65 years ago, were randomly separated into four treatment groups with different applications of moxibustion treatment. Patients were diagnosed with IBS based on Rome III diagnostic criteria. Each patient received treatment 3 days a week for the duration of 2 weeks. For each group, the scores on the Birmingham irritable bowel syndrome questionnaire, the IBS Quality of Life Scale, the Self Rating Depression Scale, the Self Rating Anxiety Scale, the Hamilton Depression Scale, and the Hamilton Anxiety Scale were measured before, during, and after treatment. Moxibustion was applied to ST25 (bilaterally) and REN6. Patients from the aconite-separated moxibustion group showed significantly lower scores after the first and second treatments. The study concluded that aconite-separated moxibustion therapy applied three times per week with one cone per application was an effective treatment for patients with IBS.

Randomized Controlled Trials (Animal Subjects)

Clinical Study #1

Han (2014) conducted a randomized controlled trial using moxibustion therapy on rats. Thirty-two Sprague-Dawley rats were randomly assigned to a blank control group (normal rats, n = 6) and a model replication (MR) group (UC rats, n = 26). A UC model was established through colonic irritation by using 2,4,6-trinitrobenzenesulfonic acid/dextran sulfate sodium enemas. Rats in the MR group were further randomly assigned to a 9-min moxibustion therapy (9M) group (9 moxa-cone, n = 6), 6-min moxibustion (6M) group (6 moxa-cone, n = 6), 3-min moxibustion (3M) group (3 moxa-cone, n = 6), and a waiting list control (WLC) group (no moxibustion treatment, n = 6). Rats in the moxibustion treatment group received 14 treatments over the course of 28 days. Moxa treatment was applied to SP15 and ST25 bilaterally. UC rats received moxibustion treatment for 3 min (3M group), 6 min (6M group), and 9 min (9M group). Three, six, and nine moxa cones were used for each treatment in the 3M, 6M and 9M groups. Colon tissue was extracted and analyzed for disease activity, colon tissue morphology, blood levels of interleukin (IL)-8 and IL-10, and the expression of Toll-like receptor (TLR)9 as well as nuclear factor (NF)-κB p65 which was assessed through disease activity index (DAI), hematoxylin and eosin staining, electron microscopy, enzyme-linked immunosorbent assay, and Western blotting. Results showed a significant reduction in DAI which indicates that moxibustion is effective in improving the disease activity of UC rats. The moxibustion treatments showed improvements in several health factors including body mass, fecal viscosity, and rectal bleeding. The comparison of DAI among moxibustion treated groups showed that the 9 min treatment gave the best improvement of disease activity.

Clinical Study #2

Zhao (2018) conducted an animal study to compare the analgesic effects between electroacupuncture (EA) and moxibustion with visceral hypersensitivity in rats with irritable bowel syndrome. Fifty 250-300 gram male rats with irritable bowel syndrome were randomly divided into four groups of ten (n=10) which received varied intensity of electrical stimulation and moxibustion heat, with a fifth untreated group that was monitored as a control group. Treatments were applied to ST37 for 10 minutes everyday for seven consecutive days. The EA stimulation frequency of 2.0 Hz was used with intensities of 1.0 mA and 3.0 mA. The moxibustion was applied at 43°C and 46°C 22mm away from the skin. Colorectal irrigation was used to induce visceral hypersensitivity and abdominal withdrawal reflex scores were taken before and after the treatments. Mast cells were taken from the intestinal mucosa and Toluidine blue staining was applied to the sample which were evaluated under a light microscope for changes. Immunohistochemical assays of intestinal mucosa was examined for expressions of 5-HT, 5-HT3R, and 5-HT4R. The results illustrated that EA and moxibustion each had greater increased stimulation effects of wide dynamic neurons in the dorsal horn of the spinal cord in model rats with visceral hypersensitivity compared to the control group. However, moxibustion treatments were found to be superior over the EA treatments. Colonic tissue mast cell degranulation rates also show significant increases in the moxibustion and EA groups compared to the control group. According to this study, the dorsal horn of the spinal cord is very important in regulating of visceral hypersensitivity and should be a therapeutic target for IBS patients. This study shows that moxibustion and EA have the potential to inhibit the response of the neurons in the dorsal horn of the spinal cord activated by visceral nociceptive afferent impulses.

Clinical Study #3

Liu (2015) conducted an animal study to measure the effects of electroacupuncture on corticotropin-releasing hormone in rats with visceral hypersensitivity. Thirty male Sprague-Dawley rats were used in the study. The rats were subjected to colorectal balloon dilation for seven weeks to induce visceral hypersensitivity. Abdominal withdrawal reflex scores were measured to assess degree of irritation as well as behavioral responses. After the initial induction of bowel irritation the rats were divided into three groups; a model group, an electroacupuncture group, and a sham acupuncture group. ST37 was used in the electroacupuncture group for its traditional therapeutic effect on the colon. Expression of CRH protein and mRNA in the colon, spinal cord, and hypothalamus were extracted and examined using immunohistochemistry (EnVision method), ELISA, and fluorescence quantitative PCR methods. Electroacupuncture was reported to significantly reduce the visceral hypersensitivity in rats and also positively modulated the expression of CRH protein and mRNA. The authors concluded that EA has the potential to play a major role in the treatment of irritable bowel syndrome.

Clinical Study #4

Weng (2015) performed an animal study to evaluate the effect of acupuncture on the purinergic receptor P2X in the peripheral nervous systems to treat the visceral pain of irritable bowel syndrome. 24 Sprague-Dawley 8 day old male neonatal rates were used in the study. The subjects were given colonic irritation through colorectal distention once daily to induce visceral hypersensitivity. The rats were divided into three groups: a normal group, a model group, and an electroacupuncture group. The electroacupuncture group was treated every day with acupuncture for seven days consecutively. The needle depth was 5mm on ST37 and ST25 bilaterally with a frequency of 2/100Hz and a current of 2 mA for 20 minutes. Abdominal withdrawal reflex scores were used to assess progress. Immunofluorescence and immunohistochemistry assays were also used to measure P2X receptor expression in the myenteric plexus neurons. Results showed that P2X expression was elevated in the subjects with IBS; however, it was downregulated in the myenteric plexus neurons after receiving EA. The EA treatments were also found to modulate the expression of P2X and its mRNA in the central nervous system. EA balanced the brain-gut neural signal transmission which gave relief of visceral hyperalgesia in the rats with IBS. The experimental results showed that the acupuncture treatments could reduce visceral hypersensitivity related IBS with a statistically significant difference.

Clinical Study #5

In 2014, Liu, Shi, and Zhu from the Department of Physiology, Medical School, at Nanchang University performed and published a randomized controlled trial to report the effect of moxibustion on visceral hyperalgesia through the P2X receptors of rat dorsal root ganglia. Forty 5-day-old neonatal male Sprague-Dawley rats were induced with visceral pain. Induction was accomplished with mechanical colorectal irritation using balloons placed into the descending colon. 60 mmHg of colorectal distention (CRD) was given starting 8-21 days after the subjects were born. Behavior responses to the CRD were examined using abdominal withdrawal reflex (AWR) scores. Moxibustion treatments started at 8 weeks in age. Rats were divided randomly into 4 groups. In the moxibustion group, UB25 was selected for treatment. Heat-sensitive moxibustion was applied for 30-60 minutes, at 2 cm over the point, for 8 consecutive days. Immunohistochemistry, RNA preparation and reverse transcriptase, and Western blotting markers were reviewed through statistical analysis ($p < 0.05$ was considered significant). Double immunofluorescence staining analysis was implemented. Results illustrated that the co-expression levels of P2X receptors were significantly increased in the moxibustion group compared to the rats in the control group. The moxibustion group observed reduced AWR scores which resulted in a therapeutic effect on the condition of IBS.

Clinical Study #6

A randomized controlled trial was performed in 2013 by Guo, Chen, and Lu. The aim of the study was to examine the effect of electroacupuncture (EA) applied to He-Mu point selections in order to reduce P2X receptor expressions in subjects with visceral hypersensitivity. A total of 32 neonatal rats were equally and randomly distributed into control, model, and electroacupuncture groups as well as a group being treated with pinaverium bromide. The rats in the electroacupuncture group were treated using ST25 and ST37. Visceral hypersensitivity was accomplished using colorectal distention and assessed with abdominal reflex scores. The group treated with electroacupuncture showed a significant reduction in abdominal reflex scores as well as comparable scores with the rats treated with pinaverium bromide. Both groups showed, through immunohistochemistry, that P2X receptor immunoreactivity was significantly lower with lowered immunoreactivity in the spinal cord. The results of the study favor the use of EA for effective treatment of patients suffering IBS.

Clinical Study #7

In 2014, Zhou, Zhao, and Wu performed a randomized controlled trial. The team started with 42 neonatal male (5 day old) rats that were screened by the Department of Laboratory Animal Science at Shanghai Medical College of Fundan

University. The rats were randomly divided into three groups: the normal group, the model group, and a moxibustion group. An IBS model was accomplished with balloons inserted 2cm into the anus and distended with 0.2 mL of air for 1 minute before. The balloon irritation was applied twice a day for 14 consecutive days. After the model was established, the rats in the moxibustion group began treatment on the 7th week. .5 cm thick moxa sticks were ignited 2 cm above ST25 and applied for 10 minutes once a day for seven days. Abdominal withdrawal reflex scores were assessed on rats within 90 minutes after the seven moxibustion treatments. Colorectal distention, using balloons, was used again for twenty seconds every four minutes and repeated five times. The results showed that AWR scores of rats at all intensities (20 mmHg, 60 mmHg, and 80 mmHg) in the moxibustion group decreased significantly. The researchers concluded that moxibustion offers therapeutic improvement to patients suffering IBS.

Clinical Study #8

Qi and Liu performed a randomized controlled trial using thermal moxibustion therapy to treat chronic visceral hyperalgesia in rats. The aim of the study was to document the relationship of moxibustion treatment to the spinal dynorphin and orphanin-FQ system. Subjects were given colorectal distention using balloons to accomplish a model of chronic visceral hyperalgesia. Male Sprague-Dawley rats began mechanical colorectal distention at 8-21 days of age. Behavioral responses were assessed using abdominal withdrawal reflex scores. At six weeks of age, moxibustion treatment was started. Moxibustion was applied bilaterally to ST25 and ST37 for 20 minutes (10 minutes for each pair of acupoints) every day for 7 consecutive days. To record the effect of moxibustion on the spinal dynorphin-k system, 3.0 nmoL/10 uL dynorphinA and 10.0 nmoL/10 uL nor-BNI were given intrathecally to the subjects 15 minutes before moxibustion therapy at the age of 43-49 days. To record the effect of moxibustion on the Orphanin-FQ receptor system, 5 ug/10 uL of Orphanin-FQ was given intrathecally to the subjects 15 minutes before moxibustion therapy at the age of 43-49 days. The expression of dynorphin and of Orphanin-FQ in the spinal dorsal horn was able to be determined by immunohistochemistry and by immunosorbent assays. Results showed levels of Orphanin-FQ and dynorphin responded positively from moxibustion treatment. Behavioral results also illustrated that moxibustion therapy significantly improved colorectal induced visceral hyperalgesia.

Clinical Study #9

Weng, Wu, and Lu performed a randomized controlled trial to measure the effect of electroacupuncture (EA) in the treatment of visceral hypersensitivity related IBS. Twenty-four 8-day-old rats were randomly divided to normal, model, and electroacupuncture groups. Colorectal distention was implemented to accomplish a rat model of chronic visceral hypersensitivity. Immunohistochemistry was used to assess P2X receptor expression in dorsal root ganglia from the study subjects. Acupuncture treatment was applied to ST25 and ST37 bilaterally. Results from the study illustrated that P2X receptors expressed in dorsal root ganglion mediated the onset of visceral hypersensitivity and that EA could reduce visceral hypersensitivity significantly.

Clinical Study #10

Liu, Zhang, Gai, and Xie performed a randomized controlled trial to identify changes in the interstitial cells of Cajal in rats with chronic psychological stress through electroacupuncture (EA) treatments on ST36. Thirty 7-week old make Wistar rats were randomly separated into a model group, an EA group, and a sham acupuncture group. Water avoidance was used as an induction technique to create a state of chronic psychological stress. Measurements and assessments were taken from diet, weight, intestinal sensitivity, interstitial cells of Cajal in the small intestine, and serum immune indexes. These measurements were taken before and after EA treatments. Abdominal withdrawal reflex scoring systems were implemented to determine visceral pain levels. Serum IgG, IgM, IL-2, and IL-6 levels were found to be significantly higher in the model group. There were no significant differences between the model group and the sham group. However, the EA group presented with the number of interstitial cells of Cajal and the synapses as significantly increased. The study concluded that, in rats with chronic psychological stress, EA at ST36 can improve food intake, weight, and reduce the symptoms of visceral hypersensitivity as well as support immune system functions.

Clinical Study #11

Wang, Zhao, Huang, and Tan performed a randomized controlled trial in order to study the effects of moxibustion treatment in the regulation of the NMDA receptor pathways in the spinal dorsal horns of rats with visceral hypersensitivity. A total of 68 newborn male specific pathogen-free 5 day old rats were used in the study. At 8 days old, the 68 neonatal rats were randomly separated into a normal group and a model group. Colorectal balloon stimulation was implemented induce a state of visceral hypersensitivity. Abdominal withdrawal reflex scores were implemented to assess pain levels. Moxibustion treatment was given perpendicularly to ST37 and ST25 everyday for seven consecutive days. Immunohistochemistry, antigen retrieval, and Western Blot samples were analyzed. After moxibustion treatment, the abdominal withdrawal reflex scores were significantly improved. Examination of the colon tissue under a light microscope illustrated that the overall structure of the colon tissues of rats in the model group was clear. There were no abnormal pathological changes such as hyperplasia, erosions, or ulcers. There was no obvious inflammatory cell infiltration and no interstitial edema. The mucosal epithelium was found to be complete and the glands of the lamina propria were found to be healthy. Detection of NR1 and NR2B in the spinal cord presented with increased expression in the model group compared to the normal group.

Moxibustion treatment was shown to both downregulate NR1 and NR2B proteins in the spinal cord. The study concluded that the expression of NR1 and NR2B protein significantly increases in the spinal cord of IBS visceral hyperalgesia rats and that moxibustion on ST25 and ST37 reverses this increase.

Case Study

Yeh and Golianu (2016) presented a case study to support integrative care treatment models in populations of children suffering gastrointestinal disorders. An eleven year-old girl was admitted to the Department of Pediatrics at Stanford University in California. Her abdominal pain was daily at a 3-4 out of 10 pain level intensity subjectively in the epigastric region. The child reported accompanying constipation lasting several days at a time with an onset several months before treatment. Her tongue was examined and revealed a thin white coat that was dry with scalloping on the sides that was puffy and pink in the tongue body. Her pulse was soft deep at the third positions bilaterally, empty in the middle right position, and wiry in the middle left position. Her diagnosis, based on Traditional Chinese Medicine, was spleen and kidney qi deficiency. ST36, LI4, SP9, SP6, PC6, and ST43 were used in the treatment with .16 x 30mm needles. After a course of acupuncture, the child felt significant improvement in symptoms. The serious limitation in this study is the fact that multiple treatment models were used concurrently.

Systematic Review and Meta-Analysis

Qin (2017) performed a systematic review titled Acupuncture for Chronic Diarrhea in Adults. The review was performed according to the Preferred Reporting Items for Systematic Reviews and Meta-Analyses Statement using the following databases: Cochrane Central Register of Controlled Trials, MEDLINE, EMBASE, China Biology Medicine disc, Wan-Fang Data, China National Knowledge Infrastructure, Citation Information by National Institute of Informatics, Oriental Medicine Advanced Searching Integrated System by Korea Institute of Oriental Medicine, and Japan Science and Technology Information Aggregator. The main outcomes measured were based on the changes in bowel movements. Secondary outcome measurements included stool consistency and quality of life scales. Other standardized rating scales were also used as well as a patient satisfaction survey and an acupuncture-related adverse effects scale. Trials included adults

18 years or older with chronic diarrhea diagnosed with functional diarrhea or IBS-D. Treatments included acupuncture, electro-acupuncture, auricular acupuncture, abdominal acupuncture, and warming acupuncture. Bowel movement changes were reported and assessed using the Bristol Stool Form Scale. Results were mixed. Some studies reported that acupuncture was more effective than sham acupuncture and some studies reported that it was not more effective. The conclusion of the review was that more Randomized Controlled Trials were needed to prove clinical effectiveness.

Chao and Zhang (2014), from the Department of Family Medicine, Sir Run Run Shaw Hospital at Zhejiang University performed a meta-analysis on the effectiveness of acupuncture in treating patients with irritable bowel syndrome. MEDLINE, PubMed, Scopus, Web of Science, and Cochrane Central Register of Controlled Trials from 1966 to February 2013 were searched for double-blind, placebo controlled trials investigating the efficacy of acupuncture in the management of irritable bowel syndrome. Studies were screened with inclusion based on randomization, controls, and measurable outcomes reported. Six clinical trials fulfilled the inclusion criteria and were used in the meta-analysis. Five articles were of high quality based on their Jadad score. The studies did not appear to cause heterogeneity in the meta-analysis. Begg's test showed P=0.707 and Egger's test showed P=0.334 which indicated no publication bias. Using the two different systems of STATA 11.0 and Revman 5.0, the authors suggested that acupuncture successfully treated the symptoms of IBS but concluded that it could not be recommended as first-line treatment due to insufficient data.

In 2013, Park, Lee, and Lee reported a systematic review and meta-analysis of twenty randomized controlled trials. Databases used were the Cochrane Register of Controlled Trials, Ovid Medline, Ovid EMBASE, AMED, the Cumulative Index to Nursing, Allied Health Literature, and China National Knowledge Infrastructure. Eight of the twenty studies illustrated that moxibustion treatment had a statistically significant outcome benefit when treating patient with IBS compared to patients treated with drug based therapies. However, there were inconsistencies among the trials. One trial showed no statistical significance in improvement after moxa treatment. 4 studies showed improvement in IBS based on global IBS symptoms when the moxa treatments were combined with acupuncture treatments. Based on another study moxa treatments did not show any significance in treatment outcomes. The authors concluded that moxibustion has a potential for improving the symptoms of IBS; however, more research is needed before it can be accepted as evidence-based medicine.

Qualitative Reviews

In 2014, Huang, Zhao, Wu, and Dou performed a literature review to evaluate the mechanisms of effect in the application of moxibustion for pain relief with patients that suffer irritable bowel syndrome. 48 research articles were reviewed based on the use of moxibustion on rats with measurable changes in secretions of the intestinal lumen and nervous system stimuli. The group concluded that mechanisms of treatment that affect IBS work on multiple organs and targets. However, quality studies were from different points of view and current systematic and comprehensive researches are still lacking.

In a 2015 review, Li and Li reported that acupuncture was effective at treating IBS and suggested a combined approach using both Western Medicine and East Asian Medical practices together in the treatment of IBS as an integrative approach. Strategies that included acupuncture produced beneficial effects with lower adverse effects and lower recurrence rates. 57 articles were reviewed, including cases studies and randomized controlled trials. Treatments included both conventional care models and AOM care models using acupuncture. The report concluded that acupuncture was effective medically, while at the same time showed reduction in cost over conventional care.

In 2014, Ma et al. performed a systematic review to assess the efficacy and mechanisms of acupuncture and moxibustion in the treatment of irritable bowel syndrome. The focus of the study was on the functions of gastrointestinal motility, visceral hypersensitivity, the brain-gut axis, the neuroendocrine system, and the immune system. In one referenced study, 10 patients with IBS-D, confirmed by ROME III diagnostic criteria, were treated with acupuncture. Acupuncture treatments showed statistically significant improvements in borborygmus frequency and colonic peristalsis. The article illustrated that acupuncture can improve colonic peristalsis in patients with IBS-D using ST36 and ST37. The authors concluded that the variety of treatment strategies using acupuncture and moxibustion make it impossible to study systematic and comprehensive issues related to the action mechanisms.

Data Summary

Figure 1 shows that that across all studies, ST36, ST37, and ST25 were the acupuncture points most often used to treat IBS. These points show the most consistent and significant improvements in the symptoms of bloat, gas, pain, Bristol Stool Scale, Anxiety and Depression scales, and QOL scales subjectively as well as the greatest measurable impact biologically based on immunohistochemistry assays, DAI scores, immunofluorescence, electron microscopy, Western blot, ELISA, Toluidine Blue Staining, and plasma sample analysis. However, it is unclear why these points were selected nor is it clear why these points are more functionally significant that other points. None of the studies discussed a biomedical rationale for point selection and none of the studies referred to a traditional theoretical framework that would support point selection. Application of moxibustion was discussed briefly as a thermal effect; however, there were no other references to biomechanics, herb properties, or even theoretical mechanisms of function aside from heat. Furthermore, the studies reviewed did not follow any consistent protocols for assessment, diagnosis, or treatment which made data comparison and evaluation difficult due to the heterogeneous nature.

Points scored

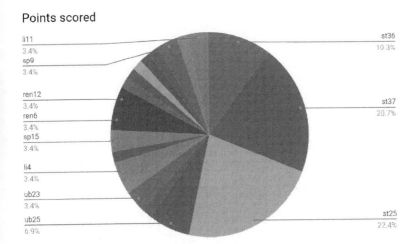

Figure 2. Heterogeneous Acupoint Usage Data

Figure 1 shows the frequency in which each acupuncture point

was utilized within all the RCT studies reviewed.

Dr. Cassone

RESULTS AND DISCUSSION

Sample sizes varied greatly between studies. The majority of the studies had sample sizes with less than 100 subjects and none of the studies had sample sizes greater than 500 subjects. Greater sample sizes produce more robust clinical trials and reviews which is a point for future research efforts to consider. The outcome measurements, which are the most important features to mark treatment success, were also highly variable. Many of the outcome measurements were subjective, which allowed for variability in interpretation. This inconsistency made the summarization of data more challenging. Table 1 shows sample size, study type, treatment, & outcome measurement.

Table 1. Sample Size, Study Type, Treatment, & Outcome Measurement

Study	Size	Study Type	Treatment	Outcome Measurements
MacPherson et al.	116	RCT	acupuncture	IBS SSS, NCSS, SF-12, PCS, MCS
Zhenzhong et al.	85	RCT	*acupuncture	VAPS, BSFS
			moxibustion	Immunohistochemistry Assay
Zheng et al.	448	RCT	*acupuncture	BSFS, SF-36
Anatasi et al.	171	RCT	acupuncture	BSFS, Rome III, CGIS
			moxibustion	bloating gas, stool pattern journals
Shi et al.	82	RCT	*acupuncture	Rome III, VAS-IBS, Immunohistochemistry
			moxibustion	
Rafiei et al.	60	RCT	catgut	Rome III, VAPS, IBS Symptoms Checklist

				Beck Depression Inventory Questionnaire
				Beck Anxiety Inventory Questionnaire
Zhu et al.	80	RCT	moxa	Birmingham IBS Symptom Scale
				IBS QOL,
				Rectal Pain Scan
Zhao et al.	166	RCT	moxa	Birmingham IBS Symptom Scale
				IBS QOL,
Han et al.	32	RCT	moxa	DAI, hematoxylin/eosin staining
				electron microscopy, enzyme-linked
				immunosorbent assay, Western blotting
Zhao et al.	50	RCT	*acupuncture	MC of colon, extracellular recordings from
			moxa	neurons in dorsal horn of spinal cord, AWR
				Toluidine Blue Staining
				Immunohistochemistry
Liu et al.	30	RCT	*acupun	AWR,

			cture	Immunohistochemistry, ELISA,
				CRH and mRNA detection in colon, spinal
				cord, and hypothalamus using QF-PCR
Weng et al.	24	RCT	*acupuncture	AWR, Immunohistochemistry, QF-PCR
				Immunofluorescence, P2X3 and RNA
				extractions from DRG and sequenced
Liu, Shi et al.	40	RCT	moxa	AWR, Immunohistochemistry,
				Immunofluorescence, P2X3 and RNA
				extractions from DRG and sequenced
				Western Blotting
Guo et al.	32	RCT	*acupuncture	Immunohistochemistry, AWR
Zhou et al.	42	RCT	moxa	AWR, QF-PCR, Immunohistochemistry
Qi et al.	n/a	RCT	moxa	AWR,

				Immunohistochemistry, ISH, ELISA
Weng et al.	24	RCT	*acupuncture	AWR, Immunohistochemistry
Liu, Zhang et al.	30	RCT	*acupuncture	AWR, IOD, ELISA
Wang, Zhao et al.	68	RCT	moxa	AWR, QF-PCR, Immunohistochemistry
				Western Blotting
Yeh et al.	1	Case Study	acupuncture	Rome III
Qin et al.		Review	acupuncture	BSFS, IBS-QOL
Huang et al.		Review	moxa	Colon mucosa and plasma sample analysis
Chao et al.		Review	acupuncture	n/a
Li and Li		Review	acupuncture	n/a
Park et al.		Review	moxa	Global IBS Symptoms, IBS SSS
Ma et al.		Review	acupuncture	Rome III, ECOM

| | | | moxa | |

In the RCTs, the details on how the treatments were performed also lacked consistency and transparency. Missing information regarding treatment strategies made it difficult to accurately compare extracted data. Many of the the studies lacked treatment details regarding needle type, needle depth, duration of treatment, or frequency of treatment. In order to build a solid case for any treatment model, the exact details of the treatments need to be disclosed. Table 2 shows treatment strategies while figure 4 shows the ratio of trials using acupuncture only, moxibustion only, and the combination of acupuncture and moxibustion.

Table 2. Treatment Strategies

Study	Point Selection	Needle Size	Depth	Tx Time	Frequency	Duration	E-Stim
MacPherson et al.					weekly	10 weeks	
Zhenzong et al.	st36,st37	.30mm X40mm	20-25mm	30 min.	daily		2 Hz/3.0 mA
Zheng et al.	st25, st37, li11	.25mm X25mm	deqi	30 min.	daily	10 weeks	15 Hz
	ub25						
Anatasi et al.	st36,st37,st25				variable	24 weeks	
	sp3, sp9, ki3						
	ki7, ub21, li11						
	liv3,ub						

	23,ub25						
	ub20,li4						
Shi et al.	st25, st37	n/a	deqi	30 min.	daily	4 weeks	2 Hz/3.0 mA
Rafiei et al.	ub17,ub23,du3	catgut				2 weeks	
	ub25,sp9,sp15						
	st25,st36,ren12						
Zhu et al.	st25, rn12,rn6				3 x/week	2 weeks	
Zhao et al.	st25, ren6				3-6 x/week		
Han et al.	sp15,st25				3 x/week	28 days	
Zhao et al.	st37	.22mm X13mm	3-5mm	10 min.	daily	7 days	1 mA/3 mA
Liu et al.	st37	.25mm X13mm	5mm	20 min.	daily	7 days	2/100 Hz

Weng et al.	st25,st37		5mm	20 min.	daily	7 days	2/100 Hz
							2 mA
Liu, Shi et al.	ub25			40 min.	4 x/day	8 days	
Guo et al.	st37,st25	.25mm X25mm	5mm	20 min.	daily	7 days	2/100 Hz
Zhou et al.	st25			10 min.	daily	7 days	
Qi et al.	st25,st37			10 min.	daily	7 days	
Weng et al.	st25,st37		5mm	20 min.	daily	7 days	2/100 Hz
							2 mA
Liu, Zhang et al.	st36		5mm	20 min.	daily	13 days	2/15 Hz
							0.1-04 mA
Wang, Zhao et al.	st25,st37			10 min.	daily	7 days	
Yeh et al.	st36,li4	.16mm X30mm					
Huang et	n/a						

al.							
Chao et al.	n/a						
Li and Li	n/a						
Park et al.	n/a						
Ma et al.	st36,st37,pc6						

Dr. Cassone

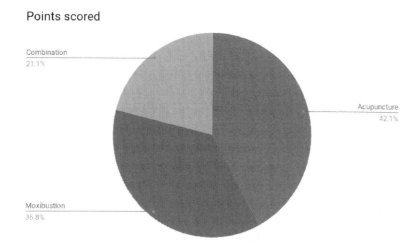

Points scored

Combination
21.1%

Acupuncture
42.1%

Moxibustion
36.8%

Figure 3. Ratio of RCTs Based on Type of Treatment

for IBS

77

The statistical significance scores provided the ability to analyse treatment models and compare effectiveness. It was established that the combination of both moxibustion and acupuncture used together outperformed the use of acupuncture and moxibustion used separately. Table 3 shows the statistical significance values for each study. Figure 4 shows the comparison of the scores based on statistical significance, sample size, quality of review, and outcomes that were considered positive.

Table 3. Statistical Significance

Study	Significance
MacPherson et al.	p<0.05 based on IBS SSS at 24 months showing no statistical improvement
Zhenzong et al.	p<0.0001 for SP expression in both Moxa and EA groups
	p<0.001 for VIP expression in both Moxa and EA groups
	showing statistical improvements in both markers
Zheng et al.	p=0.80 for stool frequency comparing EA to Loperamide
	p=0.70 for BSFS comparing EA to Loperamide
	showing no statistical difference between drug treatment and EA
Anatasi et al.	p<0.001 mean improvement covering multiple treatment strategies
	statistical improvement using acupuncture over control group
Shi et al.	p<0.01 no significant difference Moxa vs EA based VAS-IBS
	p<0.05 no significant difference Moxa vs EA based on Immunohistochemistry

	Moxa and EA equal in efficacy
Rafiei et al.	p=0.003 for pain
	p=0.002 for depression
	both p values point to signficant improvement in favor of catgut technique
Zhu et al.	p<0.01 statistical difference in improvement in IBS Symptoms and QOL
	in favor of moxa treatment
	p<0.05 statistical improvement of pain threshold upon rectal distention
Zhao et al.	p<0.001 for all criteria for the aconite separate moxa treated group
Han et al.	p<0.05 statistical significance in improvement for moxa over control
Zhao et al.	p<0.001 statistically improved over control in favor of EA and moxa
Liu et al.	p<0.01 significant CRH increase in colon, spinal cord, and hypothalamus
Weng et al.	p<0.01 statistical difference in downregulation of P2X3 in colon MP
Liu, Shi et al.	p<0.01 statistical improvement in AWR scores over control group
	p<0.01 significant reduction in P2X expression over control group

Guo et al.	p<0.01 significance in reduction of immunoreactivity in EA group
	p<0.01 significance in reduction of PK2
Qi et al.	p<0.01 significance in AWR reduction in moxa group
	p<0.05 significant improved dynorphin immunoreaction in moxa group
Weng et al.	p<0.05 significant improvment to AWR scores
	p<0.05 significant improvement in P2X expression
Liu, Zhang et al.	p<0.05 AWR significant reduction in EA group over model group
	p<0.05 significant increase in IOD of ICC
Wang, Zhao et al.	p<0.001 significant improvement in AWR for moxa group over model
	p<0.001 significant improvement in NMDA of spinal cord
Yeh et al.	n/a
Qin et al.	n/a
Huang et al.	n/a
Chao et al.	n/a
Li and Li	n/a
Park et al.	p=0.08 moxa treatments over pharmacological medications

	p=0.19 moxa plus acupuncture with improved Global IBS Symptoms
Ma et al.	p<0.05 significant improvement in borboygmus and colonic peristalsis

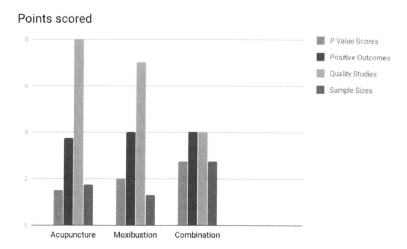

Points scored

Figure 4. Assignment of Values Based on P Values, Positive Outcomes, Quality Studies, and Sample Sizes

Figure 4 was designed based on values given to extracted data using a generalized point averaging scale. Points were awarded based on p value scores, number of outcomes that were considered positive by the authors (including subjective and objective scoring, regardless of statistical significance), number of peer reviewed RCTs, and sample sizes. Scores were tallied

and averaged based on the number of studies in each category.

ST25, ST36, ST37, and REN12 performed better for IBS related symptoms over any other acupoints used in the studies. Table 4 shows the percent to which the acupoint performance excelled. The combination of moxibustion and acupuncture is also listed as performing better when used together than when used separately.

Table 4. IBS Acupoint & Treatment Performance

treatment	comparison	improvement
acupuncture + moxa	performed separately	30%
ST25 + moxa	distal moxa	20%
ST36	chronic IBS	15%
ST37	acute IBS-D	15%
REN12	upper GI function	25%

Randomized Controlled Trials (Human Subjects)

Clinical Study #1

In the study by MacPherson et al., the main outcome measurements were based on the IBS SSS, NCSS, PCS, MCS, and the SF-12 (see Appendix A). The aim of the study was to follow up on a prior study with a 24 month post-randomization clinical trial. Two major limitations of the trial were the heavy reliance on lifestyle changes based on the initial treatments (first trial), direction given to the patients by the acupuncturists, and missing data (61% of the participants provided completed IBS SSS data). As a result, the adjusted difference between the means at 24 months was not statistically significant with the exception of NCSS and IBS SSS scores at 3 months ($p < 0.05$). The lack of statistically significant treatment effect at 24 months could be due in part to the small size of the remaining sample, and the concurrent progressive reduction in IBS symptoms in the usual care group after 12 months. The strength of this study is that it attempts to address the value of continued treatment. Since it is assumed that much of the impact of AOM treatments are cumulative, studies that assesses long term vs short term treatments are important and currently lacking. This study could be used in the future to justify maintenance programs. The weakness of this study is the declining sample size combined with high variability in treatment approaches with uncontrolled lifestyle factors.

Clinical Study #2

In the study by Zhenzhong et al., SP expression in the colonic mucosa was significantly reduced for IBS-D and IBS-C patients in both EA and Moxa groups ($p<0.0001$). There was no significant difference in outcomes between those two groups in treating IBS-D indicating that both EA and Moxa are effective treatments; however, there was a significant difference in treating patients with IBS-C. EA was more effective in reducing over-expression of SP in colonic mucosa ($p<0.024$) over moxa ($p<0.05$). VIP expression in colonic mucosa was significantly reduced ($p<0.001$) in both the moxa and EA groups after treatment. There was no significant difference between the Moxa and EA groups in treating IBS-D; however, there was a significant difference in the EA group ($p<0.001$) in treating IBS-C patients over the control group. Based on the VAPS, both the Moxa and EA groups experienced significant pain reduction from treatment ($p<0.0001$) however, the moxa group showed a significant improvement over the EA group ($p<0.001$). The authors concluded that EA and Moxa treatments were both effective in treating IBS symptoms; however, they recommend Moxa for IBS-D and EA for IBS-C. The strength of this study is the differentiation between the use of moxibustion vs acupuncture in efficacy for treating different patterns of IBS. In the future this study could be used to justify one treatment over another based on the individual needs of the patient.

Clinical Study #3

Zheng et al. divided a total of 448 participants randomly into 4 groups. 3 groups for acupuncture treatment using different acupoints and the remaining group treated with a Loperamide. There was no significant difference in stool frequency between the four groups (p=0.80) at the end of treatment and no significant difference in BSFS (p=0.07). Study showed that electroacupuncture was equivalent to Loperamide in treating IBS-D or functional diarrhea. The strength of this study is the large sample size and the comparison to drug treatment. In the future, this study may be used to justify acupuncture as an alternative treatment option over drug based treatments for IBS.

Clinical Study #4

Anatasi et al. used diagnostic patterns to decide acupoint prescriptions which let to high variation in treatment strategies and goals. The outcomes were based on reduction of pain and IBS secondary symptoms (bloating, gas, and stool consistency) that were recorded using daily journals and weekly clinical global impression scale. Overall the study showed mean statistical improvement ($p<0.001$) justifying further research (this was a pilot study). Individuated treatments decreased reproducibility and rely on practitioner experience to diagnose and select acupoints based on skill making this study less useful in a conventional care environment. This study is useful as it was one of the only studies that differentiated IBS through the AOM diagnostic patterns of IBS. In the future the eight patterns of diagnosis may be used in studies for individualized care, which is the cornerstone of AOM treatments. The weakness of this study in using diagnostic patterns is that reproducibility goes down.

Clinical Study #5

Shi et al. created their study to determine the difference in efficacy between Moxa and EA in treating patients with IBS.

Based on the VAS-IBS and immunohistochemistry assay there was no statistical significant difference ($p<0.01$ and $p<0.05$ respectively). However, they did detail a general advantage of EA in treating IBS-C and Moxa in treating IBS-D. The strength of this study is the detailed strategies using moxa and EA treatments. This study provided specific applications that will be duplicated in the future for treatment efficacy.

Clinical Study #6

The research by Rafiei et al. showed statistical significance in the areas of pain and depression in IBS patients using catgut acupuncture technique over sham acupuncture and drug-only treatments ($p=0.0003$, $P=0.0002$ respectively). Four main areas of assessment (symptoms, pain, depression, anxiety) all improved but only pain and depression showed statistical significance. The strength of this study was the prescreening of patients and exclusion of illnesses (and related medications) that could influence outcomes. It is valuable for future practices and research because the catgut technique is relatively new and there is little supportive data although the application is promising. This technique is nonexistent in the United States and, in the future, this study will help to introduce catgut acupuncture into the medical system of the United States. The weakness of this study is the number of acupoints chosen which increases variability and makes duplication difficult.

Clinical Study #7

Zhu et al. induced moxibustion analgesia in their study. Their results were in favor of moxibustion as a treatment strategy for IBS. Birmingham IBS Symptom Survey numbers along with quality of life assessments showed statistically significant improvements ($p<0.01$). The subjects were also given colorectal irritation through ballooning. The pain threshold of the moxibustion group improved significantly over the control group ($p<0.05$). In the authors' conclusion, they noted (without statistical significance) that moxibustion decreased activation of the prefrontal cortex and the anterior cingulated cortex. The strength of this study is the assessment of brain functions affected by moxibustion related to IBS. The weakness of this study is the use of an herbal barrier when applying moxibustion. The herbal barrier introduces an uncontrolled treatment variable which makes differentiation of response mechanisms difficult.

Clinical Study #8

Zhao et al. showed us that aconite-separated moxibustion group resulted in significantly lower scores (improved) (p<0.001) after the first and second treatments. The study concluded that aconite-separated moxibustion therapy applied three times per week with one cone per application was an effective treatment for patients with IBS. The aim of this study was to examine the effect of moxibustion with an herbal barrier (unlike clinical study #7). This becomes a strength as future practices may include herbal barriers when treating with moxibustion.

Randomized Controlled Trials (Animal Subjects)

Clinical Study #1

Han et al. used light and electron microscopy to show neatness of glandular arrangement in colonic mucosal epithelia. DAI has been widely used for evaluation of disease activity and allowed the integration of various aspects of disease into a single value. DAI scores were significantly improved over the control group (p<0.05) in favor of moxibustion for the treatment of IBS. Treatments were given in 3, 6, and 9 minute intervals in which the authors implied that the 9 minute treatments were more beneficial. The strength of this study is the distinction of treatment times using moxibustion. In the future, this information can be used in practice to increase efficacy based on length of time treated.

Clinical Study #2

Zhao et al. showed evidence that EA performed with different intensities on ST37 increased activation effects on WDR neurons in the dorsal horn of the spinal cord in model rats with visceral hypersensitivity at a level of statistical significance ($p<0.001$). Moxibustion treatments were found to be superior over the EA treatments. Mast cell degranulation rates in the colon were also increased in the moxibustion and EA groups compared to the control group. The dorsal horn of the spinal cord is the key to regulation of visceral hypersensitivity and it is clear, from this study, that moxibustion and EA can inhibit the response of the neurons in the dorsal horn of the spinal cord activated by visceral nociceptive afferent impulses. The strength of this study is the comparison between acupuncture and moxibustion and the outcome assessments which included the brain-gut axis. In the future this study can be used to choose either acupuncture or moxibustion based on the individual needs of the patient.

Clinical Study #3

Liu et al. performed research showing electroacupuncture was able to significantly reduce the visceral hypersensitivity in rats and regulated the expression of corticotropin-releasing hormone (CRH) protein and mRNA in the colon playing a role in the model of irritable bowel syndrome (p<0.01). The strength of this study is the examination of CRH. This outcome value is useful to support the relationship of the brain and the gut in IBS patients. This study could be used in the future to justify IBS treatments that are aimed at the brain for decrease of visceral hypersensitivity.

Clinical Study #4

Weng et al. used abdominal withdrawal reflex scores to assess progress along with immunofluorescence and immunohistochemistry to measure P2X3 receptor expression in the myenteric plexus neurons. EA showed statistical significance in improving downregulation of P2X in myenteric plexus (p<0.01). The strength of this study is the assessment of purinergic receptor function in relation to acupuncture treatments. This information can be used to justify future studies focused on the nervous system and hormone system for the treatment of IBS using acupuncture.

Clinical Study #5

Liu, Shi, et al. used immunohistochemistry, RNA preparation and reverse transcriptase, and Western blotting markers. Observations from the double immunofluorescence staining analysis showed that the co-expression levels of P2X7 receptors was significantly increased compared to the rats in the control group ($p<0.01$). The strength of this study is the examination of the DRG in outcomes. This study can be used in the future to justify further research on the nervous system for the treatment of IBS patients using moxibustion.

Clinical Study #6

Guo et al. attempted to reduce P2X4 receptor expressions in subjects with visceral hypersensitivity. After treatment, the rats from the electroacupuncture group showed a significant reduction in abdominal reflex scores ($p<.05$) and showed similar scores as the rats treated with intragastric administration of pinaverium bromide (p<.05). Immunohistochemistry revealed that P2X4 receptor immunoreactivity was significantly lower in these same two groups (p<0.01). Immunoreactivity was also shown to be lower in the spinal cord. The strength of this study is the comparison of AOM treatments to drug based treatments. In the future, this study can be used to justify giving patients an alternative to drug treatments for IBS.

Clinical Study #7

Zhou et al. performed a randomized controlled trial showing moxibustion therapy reduced AWR scores of rats at all intensities (20 mmHg, 60 mmHg, and 80 mmHg) significantly (p<0.01). They also determined the effects of moxa treatment on the expression of PK2 and showed a significant decrease (p<0.01). The strength of this study is the specificity in which the moxibustion treatments were described. The details in application, from this study, can be used in future patient care when moxibustion is indicated.

Clinical Study #8

Qi et al. performed a randomized controlled trial using warming moxibustion therapy to treat chronic visceral hyperalgesia in rats. Levels of dynorphin showed a significant response from warm moxibustion treatment ($p < 0.05$) and AWR reduced over model group ($p<0.01$). The strength of this study is the measurement outcomes based on the dynorphin system. The influence of moxa therapy on this particular mechanism of function is poorly researched. This study will allow for more research to be done in this area.

Clinical Study #9

Weng et al. used immunohistochemistry to detect P2X receptor expression in dorsal root ganglia from rats with chronic visceral hypersensitivity and recorded a statistically significant improvement over the model group ($p<0.05$). They also documented significant improvement ($p<0.05$) in AWR scores using electroacupuncture. The uniqueness and strength of this study is the specific use of ST37 and ST25, with measurable effects, on the purinergic receptor system. This is both useful clinically as well as justifies further research on this topic.

Clinical Study #10

Liu, Zhang, et al. performed a randomized controlled trial to identify changes in the interstitial cells of Cajal (ICC) in rats with chronic psychological stress through electroacupuncture treatments on ST36. They recorded significant improvements in AWR and ICC scores (p<0.05). The strength of this study is both that it incorporates psychological stress, which is an important contribution to pathogenesis, and the uniqueness of the outcome measurement of interstitial cells of Cajal. This study will support future research on both psychological and biological stress factors related to IBS.

Clinical Study #11

Wang, Zhao et al. , Huang, and Tan performed a randomized controlled trial using moxibustion therapy to treat IBS. After moxibustion treatment, the abdominal withdrawal reflex scores were significantly improved (P<0.001). Detection of NMDA in the spinal cord using western blot showed increased expression in the model group compared to the normal group (P< 0.001). Moxibustion treatment both downregulated NR1 and NR2B proteins in the spinal cord (P<0.05). These results suggest that the expression of NR1 and

NR2B protein significantly increases in the spinal cord of IBS visceral hyperalgesia rats and that moxibustion on ST25 and ST37 reverses this increase.

Case Study

Yeh et al. did a case study on the treatment of IBS in an 11 year old girl to suggest integrative care models for treatment of pediatric patients with gastrointestinal diseases and disorders. Although the patient showed clinical benefits from the acupuncture treatment there was no method for extracting statistical significance. The research team felt very strongly that acupuncture was clinically effective at treating IBS however, the acupuncture treatments were combined with dietary changes, herbal medicines, nutritional supplements, acupressure, and magnet therapies which limits the ability to gauge the efficacy of the acupuncture treatments. The weakness of this case study is that too many other modalities were combined within the treatment approach making it impossible to assign efficacy values.

Systematic Reviews and Meta-Analysis

Qin et al. performed a systematic review with mixed results were mixed. Some studies reported that acupuncture was more effective than sham acupuncture and some studies reported that it was not more effective (statistical analysis not available). The conclusion of the review was that more Randomized Controlled Trials were needed to prove clinical effectiveness.

Chao et al. performed a meta-analysis on the effectiveness of acupuncture in treating patients with irritable bowel syndrome. The analysis of six randomized controlled trials suggests that acupuncture improves the symptoms of IBS. However, the data was insufficient to recommend acupuncture as first-line treatment.

Park et al. detailed mixed results on the performance of moxa therapy as a medical treatment for IBS. While some of their reviewed studies showed statistical improvements ($p=0.08$) other studies showed no statistical improvements ($p=0.10$). The conclusion was that the authors were unable to support moxibustion as evidence-based medicine.

Qualitative Reviews

Huang et al. performed a literature review to evaluate the mechanisms of effect in the application of moxibustion for analgesia with patients that suffer irritable bowel syndrome. The group concluded that that mechanisms of treatment effects on IBS involve a number of organs and targets; however, relevant studies were from different points of view and current systematic and comprehensive research is still lacking. No data on statistical analysis is available.

Li and Li reported that acupuncture was effective at treating IBS and quoted a total effective rate at 90.48% in the acupuncture group compared to 78.95% in the medications group. The report concluded that acupuncture was effective medically while at the same time reduced in cost over conventional care; however, statistical analysis was not provided.

Ma et al. reviewed treatments that showed statistically significant improvements in borborygmus frequency and colonic peristalsis (p<0.05). These results indicated that acupuncture can immediately regulate colonic peristalsis in patients with IBS-D using ST36 and ST37. However, the authors concluded that the variety of treatment strategies using acupuncture and moxibustion make it impossible to study the complex and comprehensive issues related to the action mechanisms.

CONCLUSION

Author Opinion

In review of the articles presented in this paper, it was observed that when acupuncture and moxibustion therapies are used in combination they are 30% more effective at treating patients suffering IBS than when each of those therapies are used individually. The combination of the two treatments showed consistent improvements through both objective and subjective outcome measurements. Furthermore, moxibustion treatment showed a 20% improvement over acupuncture when applied to ST25 based on DAI scores, QOL scores, and subjective pain assessments. These subjective improvements indicate changes in the comfort level of the subjects more than functional improvements which leads the author to believe that moxibustion therapy is best applied to treat the visceral hypersensitivity and visceral hyperalgesia aspects of IBS. Although moxibustion is historically used on distal acupoints, in the treatment of IBS, moxibustion therapy is best used on local points including, but not limited to, ST25.

Another local acupoint, REN12, was not a favored acupoint for IBS treatment in the reviewed articles however, its specific use with acupuncture resulted in a 25% decrease in symptoms of the upper gastrointestinal tract such as bloat, epigastric distention, and acid reflux. These upper gastrointestinal tract symptoms are indicators of the poor digestive functions that precede the lower gastrointestinal tract irritations which ultimately result in IBS. Practitioners can approach the treatment of IBS specifically using acupuncture on REN12 with a 25% improvement to the cause and prevention of IBS over patients not treated with REN12.

ST37 showed a 15% greater improvement over ST36 when applied to patients suffering IBS-D based on the Bristol Stool Scale however, this outcome measurement is not a reliable marker for chronic corrective care. Improvements in stool pattern are desirable for the patient however, the stool pattern may worsen for a period of time while the patient's gastrointestinal irritation is actually decreasing as shown by immunohistochemistry assays. ST36 showed a 15% greater improvement regarding immunohistochemistry assays and analysis through electron microscopy. The benefit of ST37 is best observed during short term acute bowel irritation syndromes that have the symptom of diarrhea whereas ST36 has a greater overall benefit to chronic dysfunctions of the digestive tract.

Limitations in Acupuncture and Moxibustion Trials

AOM is based on a theoretical framework combined with clinical understanding, intake, and assessment while diagnosing each patient individually. Signs and symptoms give clues as to which pattern is presenting. Treatment options may vary greatly between practitioners as there is truly an art to the medicine. This fact makes AOM a challenge to study when based on Western Science parameters that focus on reproducibility in a single treatment, based on one dimensional lever systems. Individualization of treatment is a hallmark of AOM practices; however, individualization is not typically allowed in RCTs. Point selection was primarily based on Western Medical Acupuncture and AOM principles were not considered. AOM treatments usually involve lifestyle changes, dietary changes, spiritual practices, special exercises, nutritional therapies, gua sha, cupping, tui na, qi gong, herbal medicines, moxibustion, and/or acupuncture. 68% of acupuncturists treating IBS give lifestyle advice to their patients in addition to acupuncture (MacPherson, 2016). Although these practices each have therapeutic value by themselves, they are traditionally used together or in combinations to synergistically and cumulatively improve patient outcomes. In this project, only moxibustion and acupuncture were examined for efficacy in treating IBS treatment. Furthermore, IBS is a complicated disease pattern with multiple causative factors including physiological, psychological, and social contributions. There are inconsistencies in diagnosis in both Western Medical and AOM approaches. Lifestyle plays a major role in whether or not a patient improves however, not only was lifestyle medicine not used in the studies reviewed, it is impossible to control or evaluate lifestyle habits, related to pathology, in a study. Up-to-date and current studies have limited sample sizes and lack relevant medical background information on subjects that may strongly influence trial outcomes. Measurements to gauge severity of the disease and improvements were heterogeneous leading to difficulties in analyzing statistical significance. Acupuncture and moxibustion therapies are considered to have cumulative effects; however, only one of the studies investigated, by MacPherson et al., discussed continuity programs or follow up care.

Future Studies

There are many controversies regarding the use of acupuncture or moxibustion in the treatment for IBS and very few studies that show their efficacy in combination. Manheimer and colleagues reported that none of their reviewed studies found statistically significant benefits of acupuncture compared to sham acupuncture (Anastasi, McMahon, & Kim, 2009) yet many other studies, clinical reports, and thousands of years of anecdotal success support the use of both acupuncture and moxibustion applied together in treatment. In order for these AOM practices to be accepted as evidence based medicine, there needs to be a return to patient-centered or individualized care. Practitioner skill set and artistic intuitive approaches are highly valued historically in AOM practices however, these qualities are entirely discounted in the modern scientific arena. Defensive medicine, or high liability care models, have unfortunately changed the terrain of academia and scientific research. Research requires funding which can only be justified by revenue generating practices which offset liabilities. Acupuncture and moxibustion both have low direct liability in patient care (risk to benefit ratio in favor); however, there is a high liability in deviating from standard of care.

Regarding the inclusion of animal studies, although the animal study outcomes do not represent the same level clinical evidence as human study outcomes, the animal studies were included for the purpose of supporting the recommendation for future human studies.

Final Thoughts

Current medical approaches to diseases of the gastrointestinal system are costly and often involve expensive drugs or surgeries that come with serious side effects. Approaches that are cost effective with low risk or low adverse effects would serve as valuable primary or adjunct treatments to conventional care. After reviewing current research, it is the author's opinion that acupuncture and moxibustion therapies show increased treatment potential when combined together. In particular, ST37, ST25, and ST36 are the most beneficial acupuncture points in treating patients with IBS. Although the biomedical rationale for the acupoint selections was not discussed in the reviewed studies, there is support for use of these acupoints based on historical and traditional applications. ST36 is the He-Sea point of the stomach channel. The He-Sea acupoints are a subcategory of acupoints based on the five-shu division of acupoints within AOM theory. The He-Sea acupoints are known for their place on the acupuncture channels where the flow of qi goes deeper and affects the organs for which each channel is connected. In the case of ST36, the connected organ system is the stomach which directly affects functions of the gastrointestinal tract. ST36 is also grouped into the Sea of Water and Grain acupoints which are known for their influence on digestion. Historically, ST36 is used to harmonize the stomach, strengthen the spleen, and resolve dampness related to gastrointestinal tract functions. Peter Deadman, an AOM scholar, considers ST36 an essential acupoint in the treatment of any stomach fu disorder. ST37 is the lower He-Sea acupoint of the large intestine. Traditionally this point is used specifically to treat diarrhea and dysenteric disorders. It supports regulation of the spleen and stomach systems while clearing dampness which interferes with normal function. ST25 is the Front-Mu acupoint of the large intestine system. Front-Mu points are another category of acupoints that are located close to and associated with the organ being treated, in this case the large intestine. Front-Mu points are also known for their use diagnostically as they become sensitive when their related organ is in a state of dysfunction. These acupoints have been used for many thousands of years based on these theoretical assumptions and clinical reports however, supportive research describing the biomedical mechanisms of function is lacking. It is likely that the primary influence of acupuncture is neurological in effect. The response to the brain creates vasodilation to targeted tissues and organs which may involve local immune and anti-inflammatory responses. These concepts have yet to be verified scientifically.

REFERENCES

Abdullah, M., Firmansyah, M., (2013). Clinical approach and management of diarrhea. Acta Med Indones, 2013;45:157-65

Anastasi, J., McHahon, D., Kim, G., (2009). Symptom management for irritable bowel syndrome: a pilot randomized controlled trial of acupuncture/moxibustion. Gastroenterol Nurs, 32:243-55

Blackshaw, L., Brookes, S., Grundy, D., Schemann, M., (2007). Sensory transmission in the gastrointestinal tract. Neurogastroenterol Motil, 19(1):1-19

Burnstock, G., Kennedy, C., (2011). P2x receptors in health and disease. Adv Pharmacol, 61:333-372

Burnstock, G., (1997). The past, present and future of purine nucleotides as signaling molecules. Neuropharmacology, 36(9):1127-1139

Camilleri, M., Sellin, J., Barrett, K., (2016). Pathophysiology, evaluation, and management of chronic watery diarrhea. Gastroenterology, doi: 10.1053/j.gastro.2016.10.014

Chao, G., Zhang, S., (2014). Effectiveness of acupuncture to

treat irritable bowel syndrome: a meta-analysis. World J
Gastroenterol, 20(7):1871-1877, doi:
10.3748/wjg.v20.i7.1871

Chen, Y., Chen, X., Yin, X., Comparison of the therapeutic
effects of electroacupuncture and probiotics combined
with deanxit in treating diarrhea-predominant irritable
bowel syndrome, Zhongguo Zhongxiyi Jiehe Zazhi,
32:594-598, doi: 10.7661/CJIM.2012.594

Cole, S., Duncan, H., Claydon, A., Austin, D., Bowling, T.,
Silk, D., (2002). Distal colonic motor activity in four
subgroups of patients with irritable bowel syndrome.
Dig Dis Sci, 47:345-355

Dong, W., Zou, D., Li, Z., Xu, G., Zou, X., Zhu, A., Yi, N.,
Man, X., (2004). Mechanisms of visceral
hypersensitivity in patients with irritable bowel
syndrome. Zhonghua Xiaohua Zazhi, 24:8

Drossman, D., Camerilli, M., Mayer, A., whitehead, W., (2002).
AGA technical review on irritable bowel syndrome.
American Journal of Gastroenterology, 123;6:2108-2131

Drossman, D., Ringel, Y., Vogt, B., Leserman, J., Lin, W.,
Smith, J., Whitehead, W., Alterations of brain activity
associated with resolution of emotional distress and

pain in a case of severe irritable bowel syndrome.
Gastroenterology, 124:754-761, doi:
10.1053/gast.2003.50103

Elsenbruch, S., Rosenburger, C., Bingel, U., Forsting, M.,
Schedlowski, M., Gizewski, E., (2010). Patients with
irritable bowel syndrome have altered emotional
modulation of neural responses to visceral stimuli.
Gastroenterology, 139:1310-1319

Fukudo, S., Nomura, T., Muranaka, M., (1993). Brain-gut
response to stress and cholinergic stimulation in irritable
bowel syndrome. J Clin Gasterol, 17;2:133-141

Gershon, M., Tack, J., (2007). The serotonin signaling system:
from basic understanding to drug development for
functional GI disorders. Gastroenterology, 132:397-414

Giniatullin, R., Nistri, A., (2013). Desensitisation properties of
P2X3 receptors shaping pain signaling. Front Cell
Neurosci, 7:245

Grundmann, O., Yoon, S., (2014). Complementary and
alternative medicines in irritable bowel syndrome: an
integrative view. World J Gastrol, 20: 346-362, doi:
10.3748/wjg.v20.i2.346

Grundmann, O., Yoon, S., (2010). Irritable bowel syndrome:

epidemiology, diagnosis and treatment: an update for heatlh-care practitioners. J Gastroenterol Hepatol, 25:691-699

Guo, X., Chen, J., Lu., Wu, L., Weng, Z., Yang, L., Xin, Y., Lin, X., ... (2013). Electroacupuncture at he-mu points reduces p2x4 receptor expression in visceral hypersensitivity. Neural Regen Res, 8(22):2069-2077, doi: 10.3969/j.issn.1673-5374.2013.22.006

Han, Y., Ma, T., Lu, M., Ren, L., Ma, X., Bai, Z. (2014). Role of moxibustion in inflammatory responses during treatment of rat ulcerative colitis. World Journal of Gastroenterology,
20(32): 11297-11304. doi: 10.3748/wjg.v20.i32.11297

Huang, R., Zhao, J., Wu, L., Dou, C., Liu, H., Weng, Z., Lu, Y., Shi, Y., ... (2014). Mechanisms underlying the analgesic effect of moxibustion on visceral pain in irritable bowel syndrome: a review. Evidence-Based Complementary and Alternative Medicine, Article ID 895914, 7 pages, doi: 10.1155/2014/895914

Hungin, A., Whorwell, J., Tack, J., Mearin, F., (2003). The prevalence, patterns and impact of irritable bowel syndrome: an international survey of 40,000 subjects.

Alimentary Pharmacology and Therapeutics, 17:5;643-650

Ji, T., Li, X., Lin, L., (2014). An alternative to current therapies of functional dyspepsia: self-administered transcutaneous electroacupuncture improves dyspeptic symptoms. Evidence Based Complementary and Alternative Medicine, article ID 832523;7

Kanazawa, M., Hongo, M., Fukudo, S., (2011). Visceral hypersensitivity in irritable bowel syndrome. J Gastroenterol Hepatol, 26;3:119-121. doi: 10.111/j.1440-1746.2011.06640

Kang, M., Jia, H., (2008). Progress in mechanisms of visceral hypersensitivity in irritable bowel syndrome, Shijie Huaren Xiaohua Zazhi, 16(14):1554-1558

Keszthelyi, D., Troost, F., Masclee, A., (2012). Irritable bowel syndrome: methods, mechanisms, and pathophysiology. Methods to assess visceral hypersensitivity in irritable bowel syndrome, Am J Physiol Gastrointest Liver Physiol, 303(2):G141-154

Kim, D., Camilleri, M., (2000). Serotonin: a mediator of the brain-gut connection. Am J Gastroenterol, 95;10:2698-2709

Kong, F., Liu, S., Xu, C., Liu, J., Li, G., Gao, Y., Xu, H., … Tu, G., (2013). Electrophysiological studies of upregulated P2X7 receptors in rat superior
cervical ganglia after myocardial ischemic injury. Neurochem Int, 63:230-237

Larsson, M., Tillisch, K., Craif, A., Engstrom, M., Labus, J., Naliboff, B., Lundberg, P., Strom, M., Mayer, E., (2012). Brain responses to visceral stimuli reflect visceral sensitivity thresholds in patients with irritable bowel syndrome. Gastroenterology, 142:463-472

Lee, M., Kang, J., Ernst, E., (2010). Does moxibustion work? A overview of systematic reviews. BMC Res Notes, 3:284, doi:10.1186/1756-0500-3-284

Li, C., Li, S., (2015). Treatment of irritable bowel syndrome in China: a review. World J Gasteroenterol, 21(8):2315:2322

Li, S., Su, B., (2011). Irritable bowel syndrome investigation of psychological factors. Inner Magnolia Yixue Zazhi, 43:833-834

Li, Y., Zhu, B., Rong, P., (2007). Neural mechanism of acupuncture modulated gastric motility. World J Gastroenterol, 2007;13:707-16

Liu, H., Fang, X., Wu, H., Wu, L., Li, J., Weng, Z., Guo, X., Li, Y., (2015). Effects of electroacupuncture on corticotropin-releasing hormone in rats with chronic visceral hypersensitivity. World Journal of Gastroenterology, 21(23):7181-7190. doi: 10.3748/wjg.v21.i23.7181

Liu, H., Qi, L., Wang, X., (2010). Electroacupuncture at tianshu (st25) for diarrhea predominant irritable bowel syndrome using positron emission tomography changes in visceral sensation center. Neural Regen Res, 5(16):1220-1225

Liu, M., Zhang, S., Gai, Y., Xie, M., Qi, Q., (2016). Changes in the interstitial cells of cajal and immunity in chronic psychological stress rats and therapeutic effects of acupuncture at the zusanli point. Evidence Based Complementary and Alternative Medicine, Article ID 1935372, 11 pages, http://dx.doi.org/10.1155/2016/1635372

Liu, S., Shi, Q., Zhu, Q., Zou, T., Li, G., Huang, A., Wu, B., … Peng, L. (2014). P2X7 receptor of rat dorsal root ganglia is involved in the effect moxibustion on visceral

hyperalgesia. Purinergic Signaling, 11:161-169, doi:
10.1007/s11302-014-9439-y

Loguercio, S., (2012). Focus on irritable bowel syndrome. Eur
Rev Med Pharmacol Sci, 16(9): 1155-1171

Lovell, R., Ford, A., (2012). Effect of gender on prevalence of
irritable bowel syndrome in the community: a systematic
review and meta-analysis. American Journal of
Gastroenterology, 107:7;991-1000

Luo, M., He, J., Guo, Y., Li, C., Zhang, J., (2007). Effect of
electroacupuncture and moxibustion of dazhui (gv14) on
the number and distribution of degranulated
mast cells in gv14 region. Acupuncture Research, 32(5):
327-329

Ma, X., Hong, J., An, C., Zhang, D., Huang, Y., Wu, H., Zhang,
C., Meeuwsen, S., (2014). Acupuncture-moxibustion in
treating irritable bowel syndrome: how does
it work? World J Gastroenterol, 20(20): 6044-6054, doi:
10.3748/wjg.v20.i20.6044

Ma, X., Tan, L., Yang, Y., Wu, H., Jiang, B., Liu, H., Yang, L.,
(2009). Effect of electro-acupuncture on substance p, its
receptor and corticotropin-releasing hormone in rats
with irritable bowel syndrome. World J Gastroenterol,

15:5211-5217, doi: 10.3748/wjg.15.5211

MacPherson, H., Tilbrook, H., Agbedjro, D., Buckley, H., Hewitt, C., Frost, C. (2016). Acupuncture for irritable bowel syndrome: 2-year follow-up of a randomised controlled trial. Acupunct Med, 35(1), 17-23. doi:10.1136/acupmed-2015-010854

Mangel, A., Bornstein, J., Hamm, L., (2008). Clinical trial: asimadoline in the treatment of patients with irritable bowel syndrome. Aliment Pharmacol Ther, 2008;9:331-42

McFarland, L., (2008). State-of-the-art of irritable bowel syndrome and inflammatory bowel disease research. World J Gastroenterol, 14:2625-9

Mertz, H., Morgan, V., Tanner, G., Pickens, D., Price, R., Shyr, Y., Kessler, R., (2000). Regional cerebral activation in irritable bowel syndrome and control subjects with painful and nonpainful rectal distention. Gastroenterology, 118:842-848

Nozu, T., Okumura, T., (2011). Visceral sensation and irritable bowel syndrome; with special reference to comparison with functional abdominal pain syndrome. J Gastroenterol Hepatol, 26(3):122-127

Pan, G., Lu, S., Ke, M., Han, S., Guo, H., Fang, X., (2000). An epidemiological study of irritable bowel syndrome in Beijing - a stratified randomized study by clustering sampling. Zhonghua Liuxingxue Zazhi, 21:26-29

Pan, P., Guo, Y., (2009). Mast cells are one of key factors of amplifying acupuncture effect signal. Liaoning Journal of Traditional Chinese Medicine, 36(12):2066-2068

Park, J., Lee, B., Lee., H., (2013). Moxibustion in the management of irritable bowel syndrome: systematic review and meta-analysis. Complementary and Alternative Medicine, 13:247

Park, J., Rhee, H., Kim, H., (2006). Mucosal mast cell counts correlate with visceral hypersensitivity in patients with diarrhea predominant irritable bowel syndrome. Journal of Gastroenterology and Hepatology, 21(1): 71-78

Qi, L., Liu, H., Yi, T., Wu, L., Liu, X., Zhao, C., Shi, Y., Ma, X., … (2013). Warming moxibustion relieves chronic visceral hyperalgesia in rats: relations to spinal dynorphin and orphanin-fq system. Evidence-Based Complementary and Alternative Medicine, Article ID 920675, doi: org/10.1155/2013/920675

Qin, Z., Li, B., Wu, J., Tian, J., Xie, S., Mao, Z., Zhou, J., Kim,
    T., (2017). Acupuncture for chronic diarrhea in adults.
    Medicine, 96:4;e5952.
    doi.org/10.109/MD.0000000000005952

Rafiei, R., Ataie, M., Ramezani, M., Etemadi, A., Ataei, B.,
    Nikyar, H., Abdoli, S., (2014). A new acupuncture
    method for management of irritable bowel syndrome: a
    randomized double blind clinical trial. J Res Med Sci,
    19(10):913-917

Ringel, Y., Drossman, D., Turkington, T., Bradshaw, B., Hawk,
    T., Bangdiwala, S., Coleman, R., Whitehead, W., (2003).
    Regional brain activation in response to
    rectal distention in patients with irritable bowel
    syndrome and the effect of a history of abuse. Dig Dis,
    48:1774-1781

Rong, W., Spyder, K., Burnstock, G., (2002). Activation and
    sensitization of low and high threshold afferent fibers
    mediated by P2X receptors in the mouse urinary
    bladder. J Physiol, 541(Pt2):591-600

Sandler, R., Stewart, F., Liberman, J., (2010). Abdominal pain,
    bloating, and diarrhea inthe United States: prevalence
    and impact. Dig Dis Sci, 45: 1166-71

Schneider, A., Weiland, C., Enck, P., Joos, S., Streitberiger, K., Maser-Gluth, C., 2007. Neuroendocrinological effects of acupuncture treatment in patients with irritable bowel syndrome. Complement Ther Med, 15:255-63

Shi, Y., Chen, Y., Yin, X., Wang, A., Chen, X., Lu,J., 4 Rong Ji, . . .Wu, H., (2015). Electroacupuncture versus Moxibustion for Irritable Bowel Syndrome: A Randomized, Parallel-Controlled Trial. Evidence-Based Complementary and Alternative Medicine, Volume 2015, Article ID 361786, 12 pages http://dx.doi.org/10.1155/2015/361786

Shinoda, M., Feng, B., Gebhart, G., (2009). Peripheral and central P2X receptor contributions to colon mechanosensitivity and hypersensitivity in the mouse. Gastroenterology, 137(6):2096-2104

Shinoda, M., La, J., Bielefeldt, K., Gebhart, G., (2010). Altered purinergic signaling in colorectal dorsal root ganglion neurons contributes to colorectal hypersensitivity. J Neurophysiol, 104(6):3113-3123

Tamir, H., Gershon, M., (1990). Serotonin-storying secretory vesicles. Ann N Y Acad Sci, 600:53-66

Tang, Z., (2009). Traditional medicine clinical experience of the

treatment for irritable
bowel syndrome. Chin J Integr Med, 15:93-94, doi:
10.1007/s11655-009-0093-0

Wang, L., Zhao, J., Huang, R., Tan, L., Hu, H., Weng, Z., Wang,
K., Wu, H., ... (2016). Study on the mechanism
underlying the regulation of the NMDA receptor
pathway in spinal dorsal horns of visceral
hypersensitivity rats by moxibustion.
Evidence Based Complementary and Alternative
Medicine, Article ID 3174608,
11 pages, http://dx.doi.org/10.1155/2016/3174608

Weng, Z., Wu, L., Lu, Y., Wang, L., Tan, L., Dong, M., Xin, Y.,
(2013). Electroacupuncture diminishes P2X2 and P2X3
purinergic receptor expression in dorsal root ganglia of
rats with visceral hypersensitivity. Neural Regen Res,
8(9): 802-808, doi:
10.3969/j.issn.1673-5374.2013.09.004

Weng, Z., Wu, L., Zhou, C., Dou, Y., Shi, H., Wu, H., (2015).
Effect of electroacupuncture on P2X3 receptor
regulation in the peripheral and central nervous systems
of rats with visceral pain caused by irritable bowel
syndrome. Purinergic Signaling, 11:321-329. doi:

10.1007/s11302-015-9447-6

Whitehead, W., Palsson, O., (1998). Is rectal pain sensitivity a biological marker for irritable bowel syndrome: psychological influences on pain perception. Gastroenterology, 115:1263-1271

Wu, H., Jiang, B., Zhou, E., (2008). Regulatory mechanism of electroacupuncture in irritable bowel syndrome: preventing MC activation and decreasing SP VIP secretion. Dig Dis Sci, 53(6):1644-1651

Xu, G., Shenoy, M., Winston, J., (2008). P2X receptor-mediated visceral hyperalgesia in a rat model of chronic hypersensitivity. Gut, 57;9:1230-1237

Yeh, A., Golianu, B. (2014). Integrative treatment of gastrointestinal disease in children. Children, 1: 119-133. doi:10.3390/children1020119

Zhang, R., Lao, L., Ren, K., Berman, B., (2014). Mechanisms of acupuncture-electroacupuncture on persistent pain. Anesthesiology, 120;2:482-503

Zhang, N., Yu, Z., Xu, B., (2013). Research on bidirectional regulation effect of electro-acupuncture modulating jejunal motility under different conditions in rats. World Chin Med, 2013;13:255-8

Zhang, S., Li, Q., Wei, W., (2010). Consensus on standard
management of irritable bowel syndrome in TCM.
Zhonghua Zhongyiyao Zazhi, 25(7):1062-1065

Zhao, J., Li, L., Chen, L., Shi, Y., Li, Y., Shang, H., Wu, L.,
Weng, Z., Bao, C., Wu, H. (2017). Comparison of the
analgesic effects between electro-acupuncture and
moxibustion with visceral hypersensitivity rats in
irritable bowel syndrome. World J Gastroenterol,
23(16): 2928-2939. DOI: 10.3748/wjg.v23.i16.2928

Zhao, J., Wu, L., Liu, H., Hu, H., Wang, J., Huang, R., Shi, Y.,
… Tao, S., (2014). Factorial study of moxibustion in
treatment of diarrhea-predominant irritable
bowel syndrome. World J Gastroenterol,
20(37):13563-13572, doi: 10.3748/wjg.v20.i37.13563

Zhao, Z., (2008). Neural mechanism underlying acupuncture
analgesia. Prog Neurobiol, 85(4):355-375

Zheng, H., Li, Y., Zhang, W., Zeng, F., Zhou, S., Zheng, F., . .
.Zhu, W. (2016). Electroacupuncture for patients with
diarrhea predominant irritable bowel
syndrome or functional diarrhea. Medicine, 95(24):
e3884. doi.org/10.1097/MD.0000000000003884

Zhenzhong, L., Xiaojun, Y., Weijun, T., Yuehua, C., Jie, S.,

Jimeng, Z., . . .Yin, S. (2015). Comparative effect of electroacupuncture and moxibustion on the expression of substance P and vasoactive intestinal peptide in patients with irritable bowel syndrome. J Tradit Chin Med, 35(4): 402-410. Retrieved from http://www.journaltcm.com

Zhou, C., Zhao, J., Wu, L., Huang, R., Shi, Y., Wang, X., Liao, W., Hong, J., … (2014). Mild moxibustion decreases the expression of prokineticin 2 and prokineticin receptor 2 in the colon and spinal cord of rats with irritable bowel syndrome. Evidence Based Complementary and Alternative Medicine, Article 807308, 11 pages, doi: 10.1155/2014/807308

APPENDICES

Appendix A. Bristol Stool Scale

Type 1	separate hard lumps, like nuts; difficult to pass
Type 2	sausage shaped, but lumpy
Type 3	sausage shaped, but with cracks on the surface
Type 4	like an Italian sausage or snake; smooth and soft
Type 5	soft blobs with clear cut edges; easily passed
Type 6	fluffy pieces with ragged edges; mushy
Type 7	watery, no solid pieces

For IBS-D patients, the scores 4=none, 5=slight, 6=moderate, 7=severe

For IBS-C patients, the scores 4=none, 3=slight, 2=moderate, 1=severe

Appendix B. Definition of Terms

Irritable Bowel Syndrome	common condition of the lower gastrointestinal tract with symptoms
	of bloat, gas, abdominal pain, constipation, diarrhea, and sense of urgency
Visceral Hypersensitivity	increased sensitivity of the internal organs
Visceral Hyperalgesia	icreased pain of the internal organs
Substance P	a polypeptide with eleven amino-acid residues compound
	involved in the synaptic transmission of pain
Vasoactive Intestinal Peptide	a peptide hormone of 28 amino acids that is vasoactive in the intestine
Acupuncture	insertion of needle for therapeutic reponse in body
Moxibustion	application of burning mugwort to surface of body
Direct	applied directly to skin or above skin without

Moxibustion	a barrier
Indirect Moxibustion	applied with a medicinal barrier such as aconite
Electroacupuncture	electrical stimulation applied to acupuncture needles
Deqi	numbness, tingling, distention, or dull ache felt at needling site
Medical Observation Survey	quality of life assessment measuring physical functioning, role-physical
	function, bodily pain, general health, vitality, social functioning, role-
	emotional function, mental health, reported health transition
Catgut	suture made from twisted intestines of sheep

Appendix C. List of Abbreviations

IBS	Irritable Bowel Syndrome
IBS SSS	Irritable Bowel Syndrome Symptom Severity Score
SF-	Short Form Health Survey
PCS	Physical Component Sumary
MCS	Mental Component Summary
P2X	Purinergic receptor family of cation-permeable ligand-gated ion channels that open
	in response to the binding of extracellular adenosine triphosphate (ATP)
SP	Substance P
VIP	Vasoactive Intestinal Peptide
IBS-D	Irritable Bowel Syndrome Diarrhea Predominant
IBS-C	Irritable Bowel Syndrome Constipation Predominant
EA	Electroacupuncture
ATP	Adenosine Triphosphate
CRD	Colorectal Distention

VHM	Visceral Hyperalgesic Model
AWR	Abdominal Withdrawal Reflex
HSM	Heat-Sensitive Moxibustion
DRG	Dorsal Root Ganglia
PBS	Phosphate-Buffered Saline
PFA	Paraformaldehyde
GFAP	Glial Fibrillary Acidic Protein
SDS	Sodium Dodecylsulfate
HRP	Horseradish Peroxidase
SGC	Satellite Glial Cells
BSFS	Bristol Stool Form Scale
CI	Confidence Interval
FD	Functional Diarrhea
RCT	Randomized Controlled Trial
SD	Stadard Deviation
VAPS	Visual Analog Pain Scale
MOS	Medical Outcomes Survey
CGIS	Clinical Global Impression Scale
VAS-IBS	Visual Analog Scale for Irritable Bowel Syndrome
IBD	Inflammatory Bowel Disease
IBS	Irritable Bowel Syndrome Quality of Life

QOL	
SDS	Self Rating Depression Scale
SAS	Self Rating Anxiety Scale
HAMD	Hamilton Depression Scale
HAMA	Hamilton Anxiety Scale
DAI	Disease Activity Index
MR	Model Replication
MC	Mast Cell
IHC	Immunohistochemical
WDR	Wide Dynamic Range Neuron
QF-PCR	Quantitative Fluorescence-Polymerase Chain Reaction
CRH	Corticotropin-Releasing Hormone
MP	Myenteric Plexus
PKs	Prokineticins
ISH	In Situ Hybridization
IOD	Integrated Optical Density
ELISA	Enzyme-Linked Immunosorbent Assay
ICC	Interstitial Cell of Cajal
NMDA	N-methyl-D-aspartate
EC	Enterochromaffin Cells
ECOM	Electrocolonogram

ABOUT THE AUTHOR

Dr. John Cassone
MS, MSAOM, PhD, LAc, DAOM

Dr. Cassone began his career over twenty years ago using lifestyle modifications and nutritional therapies with a goal of reducing chronic illness and ultimately improving the quality of life for those he served. Today, he holds two master's degrees in health sciences, a doctorate in nutrition, and a second doctorate in integrative medicine. He has effectively treated patients from all over the world. Dr. Cassone is a board certified licensed Primary Care provider in the state of California and has published three books.

"As a scientist and a researcher, it has been my life's work to sort effectual from ineffectual treatment models. As a doctor, it is my art to investigate the complex origins of each patient's

condition and to apply techniques of corrective physiology. It is only by understanding and treating the root cause that long term health is possible." - Dr. Cassone

In 2000, Dr. Cassone opened Range of Motion, a fitness center located in San Pedro, California which has grown to become a South Bay leader in fitness & wellness. The main practice is located in Temecula, California however he is able to treat patients anywhere using modern technologies and internet conferencing.

www.drcassone.com

Contact:

Kelly Cassone, Clinical Director

info@cassonewellness.com

Made in the USA
San Bernardino, CA
21 December 2018